Perfectly Flawed

To/ Paul G,

Because :-

- you asked!

- its your birthday week

- you've been a great guy to work with ☺

Hope you Enjoy it!

Very best wishes

Clara

x

May 23rd 06

Perfectly Flawed

Molvia Maddox

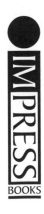

First published 2006
by Impress Books Ltd
Innovation Centre, Rennes Drive,
University of Exeter Campus, Exeter EX4 4RN

© 2006 Molvia Maddox
The right of Molvia Maddox to be identified as author of this
work has been asserted by her in accordance with the
Copyright, Designs and Patents Act 1988.

Typeset in Amasis and Folio by Keystroke, Jacaranda Lodge,
Wolverhampton
Printed and bound by Short Run Press Ltd, Exeter

All rights reserved. No part of this book may be reprinted
or reproduced or utilised in any form or by any electronic,
mechanical, or other means, now known or hereafter invented,
including photocopying and recording, or in any information
storage or retrieval system, without permission in writing from
the publishers.

British Library Cataloguing in Publication Data
A catalogue record for this book is available from the British Library

ISBN 10: 0–9547586–8–4
ISBN 13: 978–0–9547586–8–4

Cover photograph by David Peters, Wolverhampton
www.davidpetersdesign.com

I wrote this poem when my first son Nicholas was just a few weeks old. I amended the last few lines once I had my other children. It sums up how I feel about them all.

To:
Nicholas, Anthony, Krystie, Harrison and McKenna
With all my love always
Your Mom

To my son Nicholas (Because I love him)
My son as I watch you
My heart swells up with love
You are too precious
My motivation
And yet before you
I did not know, did not realise
That a person could be moved in this way
Each day you reveal a new secret
Leading me to greater heights of happiness
Thank you my son
(Thank you all my children)
Thank you for teaching me this kind of love

Contents

Preface   ix
Acknowledgements   xi

1   Lightning never strikes twice   1

2   A mother's intuition   6

3   A swimming lesson   31

4   The waiting game   34

5   Explaining 'degenerative' to a child   42

6   Reality bites   49

7   Family ties   59

8   Getting an education   69

9   Media girl   83

10 The highs and lows of 2004   90

Contents

11 What about faith?   99

12 Major surgery   108

13 Anthony's memories   127

14 The future   132

    List of useful contacts   135

Preface

Every day in the UK countless families are told that they have a child or children who have an inherited genetic condition. The repercussions of this news are like the ripples in water, they spread and grow wider and wider. As a parent you think and feel many things; often you fear that you are not normal and that perhaps you are going mad. I am writing this book as a parent who is living through this experience in the hope that in reading it, someone somewhere will know that they are not crazy; and that they are not alone.

Acknowledgements

Krystie, you inspired this book because you are the epitome of courage. You have taught me so much, I am very proud of you and I love you until it hurts.

Helen Mackleworth, thank you for reading my first few chapters and then encouraging me to carry on. Your feedback was invaluable, and your belief in this gave me the strength to finish it. xxx

Emma Wood. You know what you did! You made this happen, thank you.

Richard Willis, and everyone at Impress Books, thank you for publishing this – taking that leap of faith, honestly thank you.

Nannie Rose Dahl. Your love of books inspired me to love them too, what a blessing you gave me. I love you. You are such a truly good woman.

Mom and Dad. Steral and Molly Williams. You have stood the test of time and provided a strong framework for our family. You gave us love and guidance; you have been the very best parents, and grandparents. Do I tell you often enough that I love you because I do. Thank you both.

Karen, Mark, Andrew, Paul and Sonia my brothers and sisters. We are threaded together by our past and I love you, each of you just as you are.

Cim, my cousin who is like my sister thank you for listening.

Tracie my friend thanks.

Dr Janet Anderson and Jane Sellar. Be assured that the care and support that you continue to provide is priceless. It never seems enough to say but – thank you!

Acknowledgements

Finally Mitchell. Thank you for standing by me. It hasn't been the life we expected but we can be proud of the family that we have created. We have been blessed and I think that we are strong enough to face the future together. Love you. xxx

Lightning never strikes twice

I am an ordinary person living in the city of Wolverhampton. I have lived here all my life. My father is Jamaican and my mother is a 'Brummie'. I grew up on a council estate in the 1970s and just about remember decimalisation. I have clear memories of Edward Heath and the 3-day week. My father worked for British Rail as a trackman and financially our family struggled; but we always had wholesome food, clean clothes and a warm bed. There were four of us children; our parents loved us all; we were happy.

In December 1969 we all caught the measles; I was 7 (Mark 6, Andrew 5 and Paul 11 months). It was one of the old 'proper' winters. We didn't have central heating, just a coal fire in the front room. I remember that mom (who was always there) was keeping the coal fire burning, and because we were all poorly we were supposed to stay in the one room. Mom didn't want us to catch a chill. That was all very well, but Andrew who was just 5 was a mischief-maker. He was always laughing, such a happy soul. He was the biggest and sturdiest of us all, built like a boxer, a beautiful little boy. When the coalman knocked on the front door for his money Andrew opened the living-room door and ran to stand by our mother on the front step. I remember her ushering him back into the lounge quickly, scolding him as she led him by the hand. 'Andrew you naughty boy, you'll catch a chill, I asked you to stay in the living room, now don't follow me again.' He had that cheeky grin on his face and was giggling. Within days he became really poorly. He had indeed caught a chill.

My father played the drums in a blues/soul band at weekends. It was both a hobby and a way of earning some extra money. He usually played around the Wolverhampton and Birmingham area, so rarely went away, but that December he had arranged some gigs across one weekend in Leeds. The money was going to come in handy for Christmas so, believing that we were over the worst of the illness, my parents decided that he should keep his arrangements, and he left town for the weekend. Neither of my parents could have predicted that Andrew would take a turn for the worse, but he did. I can still remember vividly that Andrew got really poorly; he had a fever and was very hot. He couldn't quite catch his breath; his breathing was really laboured.

My mother came from a small family; she only had one brother and was the youngest child. She didn't have lots of experience with children. My father, on the other hand, was the second eldest of eleven. He had helped his mother with his younger siblings, nursing them through many illnesses, and was very natural when it came to looking after sick children. Nothing fazed him; he had actually delivered Andrew when mom went into labour unexpectedly, so he felt a strong bond with him. My father was quite 'instinctive', and just always seemed to know what to do. My mother relied on him a lot. Now that Andrew was so poorly, she didn't really know what to do. You must remember that people were not well informed back then, as there just wasn't the access to information that we have today. We didn't have a telephone at home so mom went down to the telephone box and called the doctor. She explained that she couldn't bring Andrew to the surgery because he was too ill and requested a home visit. Later that evening, some time after six o'clock, the doctor arrived. Mom was explaining the problem as they walked from the front door into the living room. I remember the scene as if it were yesterday. He bustled in, put his bag on our dining table, which was against the back wall. He got out his prescription pad and started to write. All the time he was moaning that it was late, and that he hadn't had his tea. He never once actually went over to Andrew, who was propped up in an armchair wrapped in a blanket in front of a roaring fire, clearly struggling to breathe. If only he had listened to Andrew's chest, things would have been different I'm sure. He gave mom the prescription and left. She was really worried, but she hated being a nuisance. She kept Andrew warm. He was sitting directly in front of a roaring coal fire (the exact opposite of what you should do!), and she sponged him down every couple of hours, but he kept getting worse. Later that night when we were all in bed, mom got really concerned about Andrew. He was sleeping with her, so that she could watch him. She really didn't like the sound of his breathing and ran to a neighbour's house to use the telephone. She called an ambulance, and Andrew was rushed to hospital. Andrew had developed pneumonia and now became unconcious, his life ebbing away. The doctors resuscitated him, and put him on a life support machine.

The police contacted my father up in Leeds, but somehow got the message confused, and so told him that it was my mother who had died. He collapsed in shock, and kept asking them if they were sure. He explained that his children had measles but were not too bad when he left home; but his wife had been absolutely fine, so he couldn't understand what had gone wrong. The band travelled back to Wolverhampton, and as they pulled up at the hospital he saw my mom standing on the hospital steps. She had left Andrew to get some air. She explained what had happened and they went back to discuss Andrew with the doctors. After four days they agreed to turn off his life support machine. Andrew died on 16 December 1970.

The shock to our family was terrible; it was such a sad time. I grew up overnight; my safe world shattered. I learnt that life can be cruel and that the unexpected can and does happen. It took away my innocence.

Mom was not herself for a long time. She 'fretted' and became nervous, the grief engulfed her really. Part of the reason that my mom was so distressed was that unbeknown to us she had another daughter, Karen.

Mom was unmarried when she fell pregnant with Karen, and, furthermore, Karen's father was black. In the early 1960s this was considered to be a terrible thing. Mom was sent away to a mother and baby home to give birth, and she was supposed to give her baby up for adoption once it arrived. However, once she had delivered Karen and seen her, and held her, she couldn't do it. So she returned home to Birmingham taking Karen with her. She went back to her parents, who helped her to bring Karen up. Unfortunately for many reasons, but mainly the feeling of shame, my grandparents told the neighbours that they had fostered Karen. Once the lies started they never stopped. Karen was brought up as my grandmother's child. My mom was only 18 herself, and was very upset about everything. She moved to Wolverhampton when Karen was about 6 months old with the intention of sorting out her life and creating a home in which to bring up Karen herself. But sadly this never came to be. Mom met my father and told him about Karen; he was more than willing to bring Karen up as his own. But by this time Karen had been with my grandparents for many months. They absolutely adored her and understandably didn't want to give her up. So it was never resolved and Karen stayed with my grandparents. The whole situation was cloaked in great secrecy. We knew Karen, and she knew us, but we were told that she was mom's adopted sister. We loved Karen and spent school holidays together, but we didn't realise that she was actually our own sister. None of us children were told the truth until Karen was 15 and I was 13. So you see, at the time of Andrew's death, my mom felt that she had lost two children: Andrew because of sickness, and Karen because she had not been strong enough to stand up for her and claim her as her own. My mother's unresolved grief and disappointment in herself over the way that she had lost Karen merged with the grief of losing Andrew and plunged her into deep depression.

We children just got on with things. We were sad, but children don't dwell on things, and think their thoughts on their own. I remember feeling very sad some days, but, on the whole, life just carried on. I became a real little helper getting on with chores. Mom wasn't herself, so I felt responsible for helping to keep things going. I wasn't asked to do it, but I just did. Mom, who was understandably upset, needed the support. I think that all of this made me a 'coper' and an organiser. We talk about it now, and she says that she was on the edge of a nervous breakdown. She says that for a long long time, she felt that she wanted to curl up in a ball and shut the world out. She would imagine that someone would knock on the door one day to tell her that there had been a big mistake and that Andrew was alive. She just could not accept his death, so she would do little, strange, forgetful things like buying four packets of sweets. Often she served up Andrew's dinner only to remember as she brought the plates to the table that he had gone. She had a picture of Andrew, Mark and I together, and she carried it everywhere with her, because she just felt that she had to have him with her all of the time. She just didn't feel right with only three children at home, so my parents went on to have another baby: my youngest sister Sonia. I was 10 when she was born, and we were all delighted. She gave mom a new lease of life and put her on the road to recovery. My father got a better-paid job at a foundry casting metal car parts, and we moved to a 'bought' house. But oh, what a tangled web we weave! Eventually the truth about Karen and the fact that she was our sister came out. It was a shock, but a pleasant one. I was pleased to know that I had an older sister. Karen stayed with my grandmother, but most holidays she either came to us, or Mark or I went over to her home. She felt like our sister, and always has. Karen had to come to terms with the revelation, and my mother had to overcome her feelings of guilt. But it was all just so long ago and times were very different. It was a further sadness to know that we didn't all grow up together, but we are not the first family to experience such a situation and we won't be the last. In spite of everything you do get back to normality, life does go on.

When I married and had my own children, I always had an unexplainable fear or dread at the back of my mind. I had a feeling that something bad was going to happen and that one of my children would die. For each of them I have dreaded their fifth year, and been so relieved once they have reached their sixth birthday. I always felt that Andrew's death had left me hypersensitive. I told myself not to worry, and pushed the niggling fear to the back of my mind; after all, lightning never strikes twice, does it?

A mother's intuition

2

Much has been written about a mother's intuition. When you talk to women about it, most can relate an example of a sixth sense that kicks in. However, it is also true that women often 'tune it out'. It doesn't seem rational, so sometimes we choose not to trust it.

My strange feeling never really went away. It hung about in the back of my mind, a feeling of panic that stayed just below the surface. Over the years things happened, but then situations resolved. I scolded myself, convinced that my brother's early death had affected my nerves and given me these ridiculous fears. Now I look back and wonder. Let me explain.

I really do feel that I have been blessed. I have five children: Nicholas, Anthony, Krystie, Harrison and McKenna. More than anything else that I have done in my life they are my greatest achievements. I am not an 'earth mother' type, but I have strived to teach my children well, and enjoy them. I have valued them as little people, and been grateful that they have kept me grounded and reminded me of the simple things in life. I have enjoyed discovering the world through a child's eyes five times over! The simple things like watching a ladybird climb a stem of grass, or wondering at a magnificent spider's web with a million raindrop diamonds glistening after the rain. Collecting blackberries, baking cakes, rolling down hills and chasing the waves into the sea. Reading my favourite poetry with them, singing along to the radio in the car at the top of our voices, and playing mad games on rainy days. Yes I have been blessed.

I have been married twice. I married the first time when I was just 18. At 20 I had my first son Nicholas, quickly followed by Anthony two years later. I loved my boys. However, during both of my pregnancies I had desperately wanted a girl. Both times whilst I carried them I had visions of a little girl called Sophie Elizabeth. I didn't get my Sophie Elizabeth, I got a Nicholas and an Anthony, but once I saw those little faces and held those tiny bundles I just loved them, 'My boys'.

We had a happy life, and together with my first husband we worked hard. We built a nice home together and had a nice lifestyle. But I still had that niggling fear at the back of my mind. It haunted me silently.

When Anthony was about 7 months old, my brother-in-law dropped him. We were visiting, and my brother-in-law stood over by his fireplace. Anthony was sitting on his arm; he had his back to the room, and was facing his uncle. He was laughing at him. As they played with each other, he was getting excited as babies do and started to 'bob' up and down on his uncle's arm in a bouncing motion. My brother-in-law didn't have children, and must have thought that he was holding Anthony securely. He didn't use his other hand to steady the baby's back as a parent would. Anthony got so excited that he suddenly pushed back off his uncle's chest and simply toppled over his arm and crashed to the floor. He missed the fireplace by less than a couple of inches. Everyone froze in horror. I clicked into autopilot and ran over to pick Anthony up off the floor. Anthony wasn't crying. 'He's alright,' I said, 'look he's not crying.' I cradled him to my chest, and then cupping his head in my hands I tipped him away from me to check his face. He had watery, slightly blood-stained fluid coming from his ear. It had stained my shirt. I looked at this in horror. 'Oh my goodness he's leaking his brain fluid' I said. I thrust him into his father's arms, and ran out of the room. Everyone else in the room was still frozen and fairly quiet. I knew that my in-laws didn't have a house phone, so I ran for the front door, out along the footpath and round to the neighbour's house. I hammered on the door. As soon as the neighbour opened it, I pushed him out of the way. I was clearly distressed, and shouted at him, 'I'm sorry but I need your phone, my brother-in-law has dropped my baby and we need an ambulance.' The man stood back and pointed to the phone in the hallway, but I already had it and was dialling for an ambulance. I gave our address details, thanked the man and ran back to the house. When I ran into the lounge everyone was still just standing in shock, they didn't know what to do. I looked at my husband to see that Anthony was going to sleep; I snatched him away from his father. 'He mustn't go to sleep,' I shouted, 'He mustn't.' I took him out into the cool evening air, and stood on the front lawn gently patting his very dopey face. I felt sick with fear. 'No Anthony please don't go to sleep, come on baby, stay awake. Anthony, baby, mommy's here. Please don't die.' I paced up and down patting him gently, talking to him, willing him to live. In the back of my mind, I kept thinking that this was my fear, this was what I had been expecting, the loss was going to happen now. I shouted back to my family who were stood around the front door watching me, 'Where is the ambulance, where are they?'

The next thing I knew the ambulance arrived. I remember the paramedic taking Anthony from me as we climbed into the back. My husband came with me. I looked over at Nicholas's concerned little face as he stood with his uncle; he was only a baby himself, not even 3. The doors shut, and we sped out of the close. I felt relieved that help had arrived, and I kept watching Anthony as we drove through the streets towards the hospital. After a few minutes I remember turning to my husband to say, 'It can't be too bad, because they haven't got the blue lights on.' Just as I said this, Anthony started to vomit. He was a baby, 7 months old, purely breast fed, and yet in just over a minute he half-filled a bucket with vomit. The paramedic didn't say anything to us; he just leaned forward, tapped the glass between us and the driver, muttered something and the blue lights went on; the driver put his foot down and we flew the rest of the journey to the hospital.

As soon as we pulled up, the doors crashed open and Anthony was taken away on a stretcher. I was watching him intently, but out of the corner of my eye I saw two police officers. I noticed that the paramedic went to talk to them, he was shaking his head, the officers looked over to my husband and me and then walked away. I knew straight away that the paramedic was telling the police that we hadn't harmed our child, this wasn't an abuse case. I remember thinking how quickly the wheels of 'big brother' click into motion.

I ran into the hospital. 'Where is he? Where is my baby?' I shouted. A nurse approached and started to ask me questions as she ushered us into a cubicle and drew the curtains; name, age, date of birth. I answered her, then suddenly said, 'Stop asking me stupid questions. Where is my baby?' She said that she needed to fill a form in. I looked at her, stood up, marched out of the cubicle and shouted to some people sitting down,

'Where did they take my baby? Did you see a baby?' A woman pointed down the corridor, 'They took him in there love.' I ran to the curtains that she pointed out, and a doctor quickly took my arm and led me into another cubicle. I sat down, and they started the questions again. I tried to answer and then the frustration grew. I shouted, 'I am not sitting in here while my baby is out there.' I ran out of the cubicle and into the area where they were looking at my Anthony. I shouted defiantly as I burst in, 'He is my baby and I am not leaving him.' I saw a doctor nod to the nurse who was approaching me; he was signalling to let me stay. I went and stood by my baby and talked gently to him. I looked at the nurse and said, 'What ever you need to do, you do it with me next to him.' They took us into an X-ray room, and I held him in position on the X-ray table as they took the necessary photos. They did lots of tests and over the next couple of hours it became apparent that he was not seriously injured. He stayed in hospital for two days, and then he was discharged with follow-up outpatient appointments. He held his neck bent over to the left for about two to three months after the accident, but eventually made a recovery. He didn't seem to have any lasting damage. However, a few years later, when he was 4, we found out that he had in fact damaged his hearing, and was nearly totally deaf in his left ear. But when you consider how close he was to the actual brick fire hearth itself, less than two inches, he was incredibly lucky. Things could have been a lot worse. I thought that maybe this was the 'doom' I had been expecting, but the fear remained; it just wouldn't go away.

Actually Anthony was to provide us with another drama a few years later. He was rushed into hospital with appendicitis, but he came through it. The boys grew older and stronger, and we were all content with our lot.

I kept a dream in my mind that at some point in the future I would complete our family with a little girl. I even bought a book entitled, 'How to choose the sex of your child by diet'. I remember reading it and noticing that the foods on the boy diet were the foods I naturally ate, so I decided to change my diet to include the 'girl' foods. Even though I didn't intend to have a baby yet, I reasoned that I might as well alter the chemical balances in my body as soon as possible. At 28 I was shocked to find that I was pregnant again. I didn't know how to feel. Part of me was happy, part of me was sad. I liked our life and didn't really want to change things. I also had this feeling that I hadn't done everything that I

9

had wanted to do to ensure (as far as you can do) a little girl. I was quite depressed about the pregnancy. I didn't want to tell people, and it took me about five months to come to terms with it. At the same time I felt really guilty because I wasn't overjoyed. I felt that I was short-changing the child that I was carrying. To make matters worse I felt really ill.

I hadn't carried my boys particularly well. I suffered with frequent daily bouts of vomiting. The sickness lasted for the entire pregnancies. I developed pre-eclampsia with both of them, spending lots of time in hospital on bed rest. I definitely didn't bloom. However, both of my births were fine (if a little quick). I used to tell myself that you couldn't have it both ways, but wondered why so many of my friends seemed to feel quite well.

Now here I was again, constantly sick, always tired. I felt dizzy and unable to cope with a normal day's activities. I remember asking a doctor why I felt so sick during my pregnancies. He said he couldn't really say, but that maybe my hormone levels were high. He also made a comment about the genetic mix. This comment always stayed with me and I wondered about it a lot. He said that sometimes the genetic mix of the mother and father isn't good and that might account for the sickness. At the time I remember thinking about my boys and how beautiful they were. I remember thinking that his comment was completely ridiculous, but even as I thought that, I buried the comment in my memory. It was a memory that hurtled to the forefront of my mind just a few years later.

The pregnancy developed, events taking their usual course. I got used to the fact that our family would be growing and I was happy again. I continued to be sick and feel unwell, but finally the day came when I knew that my labour had started. I went along to the hospital with her dad and expected everything to go to plan. But it didn't. I was of course taken to a delivery suite and strapped up to the obligatory monitor, but it wasn't registering my contractions. First a midwife examined me, and then a doctor, but no one could tell that I was in labour. I felt really surprised, because as far as I was concerned everything felt normal to me. I could definitely feel the pain and the tightening, but no, the general opinion was that I had a water infection and was not in labour. I began to get visibly upset, and I begged the doctor to fetch my notes and read what happened when I had last given birth to Anthony, because he had surprised the medical staff by arriving much, much faster than they had anticipated. Then, as now, I had been sure that the baby's arrival was imminent, but they wouldn't listen. The doctor (a woman) did eventually fetch my notes and stood in front of me and read them, but then said, 'No, this time it's different, you are not in labour, I'm going to send you back to the ward with some painkillers for a water infection.' I was in shock. I started to sob quietly, I could hardly talk, but I took her hand and started to ask her to really check that I wasn't in labour. Every word was broken by sobs, I could barely talk, but I remember asking her to please perform a section and get my child out if necessary. 'This pain that I am feeling is definitely labour,' I said, 'but if you are telling me that I am not dilating, then my body is not working properly, and I am scared about what will happen to this baby because it wants to be born now.' The doctor looked at me very kindly and told me not to worry, and then sent me to the ward. By now it was eleven o'clock at night, and I was tired, upset and defeated. I remember saying to my husband that we had done everything that we could possibly do, but if our child was stuck, and if she died, we could do no more. We were both upset, but he decided to go home to get some rest. I went to the toilet, and then got back into bed. I prayed really hard, and then went to sleep. Ten minutes later I was woken by the strongest urge to push. It was less than half an hour since I had been sent to the ward. My husband had only left me fifteen minutes ago. I rang the bell. The midwife came, and was very 'off' with me. 'What do you want Mrs Lue?' she asked. 'I need to push,' I replied. She rolled her eyes and said that she would need to fetch some gloves. I very calmly waited as I carried out my breathing techniques. She didn't rush, and after about five minutes came back. She lifted the blanket off my bed and prepared to examine me, and then said 'Oh my God', as she rang the bell, and said, 'Hang on Mrs Lue, don't push yet, let's get you to delivery.' I begged her to phone my husband and get him back to the hospital. It was about 11.25 p.m. by now, and everyone was rushing around. They couldn't get a porter to move my bed, so they put me in a wheelchair and started to push me to the lifts. All the time, I was breathing like mad, because the pains were so strong, and I really wanted to push. Then I started to shake. It was almost like someone had run electrical power lines through my body, the whole of my being was shaking so violently. Eventually the midwives decided to push me up to delivery themselves. At about 11.40 I was taken to a delivery suite. The midwife was asking me to hang on while they prepared the room. I was lying on a bed shaking like mad, and trying to keep calm by breathing. I was desperate for my husband to get back, so was fighting the urge to push as much as I could. I remember using the gas and air, and breathing really hard, then the sound of doors crashing as my husband rushed in. It was about 11.55 now, and the midwife finally said that I could push. However, I had spent that long holding it, that I was scared now, and I remember asking her, 'Are you sure I can push, am I dilated properly, I won't tear will I?' How strange! She half laughed, and said 'You've spent the last half an hour telling us you wanted to push, now you can.' So I did. And that's literally all it took, one push. My husband said it was so fast that the baby almost flew out; it was 12.05, just turned midnight. As soon as she was born the shaking that had calmed down began again, and I was once again convulsing so violently that my body was jumping up and down on the bed. I asked through chattering teeth what was wrong with me, and the midwives told me that I was in shock. The doctor who had seen me just a couple of hours earlier came to visit me. She knelt down at the side of the bed, took my hand and squeezed it tight. 'I'm so sorry,' she said, 'but we couldn't tell. You have had a precipitate birth, which means that we couldn't know that you were in labour, only you would know. Next time you have a baby, you must tell them about this.' I was still shaking, and through chattering teeth, I said, 'but I did tell you, I asked you to read my notes about Anthony, because he was a bit like this, not quite so bad, but similar.' 'I know,' she said, 'I'm sorry.' She had tears in her eyes. I looked at her, and said, 'After tonight, I will never ever have another baby, I couldn't take it.' So that was it, 28th March 1990, Krystie Rosa Elizabeth arrived (I had decided not to use the name Sophie!). I was ecstatic. My much longed for daughter had arrived.

That night I was taken back to the ward and eventually went to sleep. At about 3.30 a.m. I woke up again shaking violently from head to foot. My whole body once again jumping on and off the bed. I rang the bell, because I felt really scared; a nurse came to me, and told me that I was in shock. It was horrible, and unbeknown to me was to cause me medical problems over the next few years.

I loved Krystie the minute I saw her; she was beautiful, a lovely baby. She was also pleasant and good-natured. She reached all her milestones either slightly early or just about on time. She was a stubborn little miss, a bundle of energy and very loving. Dainty and petite, the girl that I had imagined. *I thought she was perfect.*

However, I developed post-natal depression. I didn't realise for a long time, though the signs were there. I never once rejected Krystie, but I couldn't cope with my own life. I remember being terrified of getting pregnant, so my husband agreed to have a vasectomy. I just couldn't face the thought of going through that birth experience again. I had felt helpless that night because I knew that I was in labour, and yet everyone was telling me that I wasn't. I thought that my body had got stuck, and that my child would die inside me. Even now, it upsets me to think about it.

My mind didn't work properly. I found everything too much. My mind couldn't organise anything. From the time I got up in the morning until I went to bed at night everything seemed too much. I looked after the children, they were clean, well dressed and fed, but it was everything else. For example I would get back from the school in the morning and think, Molvia wash the breakfast things up. I would start the washing up, and part way through think, 'Oh no, I never made the beds!' I would leave the washing up unfinished and rush off to make the beds. Part way through this task, I would think, 'Molvia put the washing on'. I would leave the beds half done to sort the washing, and part way through this remember the washing up. I spent my days going round in circles, not achieving anything. My once orderly house descended into chaos.

I remember telephoning the school in tears to say that the boys were going to be late. This happened several times. On another occasion I remember telephoning my mother-in-law in a panic asking her to please come and take my boys to school for me. One morning I got back from the school run, and just collapsed in a heap. I telephoned the doctors surgery and begged the receptionist to send my doctor out to me. Thankfully my doctor knew me very well. He came at the end of his morning surgery. He was so kind, he sat and talked to me, and listened to how I felt. He said that I was depressed and offered me tablets. He explained that sometimes nerves need a bandage and that I should use the tablets like that bandage. This was very hard for me. I was Molvia, the strong organised woman who managed everything. I accepted the prescription and fetched the tablets but only took them for a few days. (Strong Molvia didn't need tablets – but I kept the boxes in the cupboard just in case, and took them occasionally just a few days at a time.) Consequently I got worse. I had taken extended unpaid maternity leave from my job, but when it was time for me to return to work, I couldn't. I tried, but I couldn't remember how to do anything, even processes that

I had designed seemed alien. I couldn't remember how to use the computer, and I had to go on sick leave. I kept visiting my doctor, though, and because I had some other strange symptoms (I had gained 3 stone in weight, and my periods suddenly just stopped) he took blood tests and found a problem. He referred me back to my obstetric gynaecologist. Eventually it transpired that I had an underlying problem that had been brought on by the shock that I suffered at Krystie's delivery. The precipitate birth (which means very fast) had caused problems with the pituitary gland, which manages the endocrine system. My whole hormonal system was unbalanced, and this had affected my nerves and caused other problems, such as the weight gain and erratic periods. I was under the hospital as an outpatient for many months; looking back, I do not know how I coped, because I felt so ill. Every day was like being in a dream, like I was fighting for air. Everything seemed too hard, and I just couldn't cope. I was given hormone replacement therapy, finally being discharged when Krystie was just over 2 years old. My husband's life seemed to carry on as normal: he went to work, played his sports, etc. I felt like I was on my own, just struggling to get through each day. I loved my children, and I never ever neglected them. I was still very loving to them, and patient with them, but our home was disorganised and I couldn't seem to cope. This made me feel even worse. I had always been so house proud. I remember a friend saying to me once that she felt like she could eat off my floor, everything was so immaculate. That's how I like things to be, so the fact that I wasn't sorting things out made me feel even worse.

During this time we had another traumatic experience involving Anthony. He developed a cough that just wouldn't go away. I had taken him to the doctors about three times over a period of weeks, but nothing shifted it. One Thursday evening we had gone out, and Anthony was complaining that his left arm was really hurting him, right up into his shoulder. When we got back home, he really didn't look well, so we put the other two children to bed. We had tucked Anthony into bed too, but at the last minute I decided that he would be best resting on the sofa with us in the lounge so that we could watch him. His father carried him downstairs and laid him down. I walked in to the lounge to see his eyes rolling back in his head; all you could see was the whites of his eyes and his breathing was laboured. I screamed out for my husband to come quickly. Looking at Anthony all I could see was my brother Andrew and his struggling to breathe. I was shouting, 'Its like Andrew; it's just like

Andrew!' Fortunately his father was trained in first aid; he calmly altered Anthony's position so that he was propped up on cushions instead of lying flat. Then he looked at Anthony and said, 'Look son, look at daddy, don't panic. I want you to breathe when I say. Are you listening?' Anthony nodded. With that he simply sat and said, 'Breathe in, breathe out, breathe in, breathe out', and Anthony watched his father, and breathed when he was asked to. I meanwhile called a doctor. When she arrived, she called an ambulance and once again he was taken to hospital. I sat with him during the journey; that feeling of fear again, especially since he had brought all of the memories of Andrew flooding back. Once we arrived at the hospital they examined him, X-rayed his chest and told me that he too had pneumonia, so a few days in hospital on strong antibiotics restored his health. We had already booked a holiday to Almeria in Spain, so it worked out that we flew out to Spain just a few days after he was discharged. The consultant felt that the warm sunshine would do Andrew the world of good. I remember starting that holiday believing that someone was definitely looking after us.

We had a really nice holiday, but during the second week of our stay, an incident occurred that gripped us all with fear. We had gone on holiday with my parents, my younger sister and her boyfriend, and my brother and his wife. My nerves were still weak; the stress of Anthony being in hospital was still hanging over me and my husband and so we had been bickering. The whole family decided to go for a walk to the beach. I had left the garden of our apartment, and various members of our group followed the boys and me into the quiet back road. I was engaged in some banter with my father when we both noticed that Krystie had wandered away from our group and was heading up the road away from us. She wasn't quite 2, and looked like a walking doll. Her father was closer to her than me, so I shouted to him to get her, but he was a bit annoyed with me because we had been bickering, so replied that I should get her myself. My father was saying that he felt a little girl shouldn't be allowed to wander on her own, and I was begging Krystie's father to fetch her. 'Come on,' I said, 'you're much closer than me, please just grab her.' Suddenly he turned tail, and started walking quickly towards her. In that same instant, we all heard the revving noise of a car approaching us. We couldn't see the car, but we could hear it gaining speed, and we all knew that it was heading for Krystie. My husband had broken into a quick jog and my brother now began to rush toward Krystie. The car appeared just as her father scooped her up. He lifted her and instinctively turned his back to the car. The car driver having caught sight of them, began to perform an emergency stop. As the car skidded trying to avoid them, the tyres screamed, and the grit from the road churned up a dusty white cloud. The car came to a stand-still, with just an inch between its bumper and the back of my husband's knee. Our group was a mixture of startled faces, covered eyes, screams, shouts and sheer horror. My father was looking on in disbelief. 'Good God again,' he said, 'I thought we were going to be taking Krystie home in a coffin.' I could hardly breathe, whereas my husband was breathing heavily. Krystie was crying. I was so glad that my husband had stopped arguing with me, and just turned to get her, because if he had not already been on the path towards her, that car would have definitely hit her. Its bumper would have hit her forehead, and she would not have survived.

The Spanish car driver was in shock; he shook his head and was apologising profusely. Yes he had been driving far too quickly, but we apologised too because we should not have let her wander off, even if it was only a matter of a few feet in a quiet back lane. He continued on his way, and we walked fairly quietly down the lane. As we turned the corner, we saw the young man, stood at the side of his car; he had obviously reached his house. His eyes closed in sheer thankfulness; he was clutching his own daughter, who looked a similar age to our Krystie, tightly to his chest. He held her for several minutes. When he opened his eyes, we were walking past him, and he nodded to us; we nodded in reply back to him. He was as white as a sheet and clearly very upset at what might have been. My heart was once again strangled with fear; I had a feeling that we had escaped another drama. Surely that was it; surely nothing else could happen to us ever again.

My illness had put a terrible strain on my marriage. Looking back, I can see now that my husband just couldn't understand why his rational, very capable wife just couldn't seem to function. For my part I couldn't understand why he didn't understand my problem, and support me in a stronger way. A massive gulf developed between us. We separated when Krystie was about 2½, and divorced just over a year later.

I felt that my divorce was a terrible thing. Even though I thought that it was the best thing for us as a couple, I felt a failure. It was upsetting for everyone involved, not just the children, my husband and me, but also for our families. We had been married for twelve years when we separated. To outsiders we had the perfect marriage and life. I know from experience that people are very good at presenting a brave face to the outside world. I personally had not felt able to admit when I was struggling, and consequently people didn't realise. Therefore to outsiders the shock of our separation was worse.

All of this happened in the early 1990s. Everyday when I opened my newspaper there was another article blaming the ills of the world on single parents. Everything I read seemed to indicate that our children would be psychologically damaged. I had visions of my boys ending up in prison, blaming their demise on me. In reality, though, we had been a strong family unit with strong values. Those values didn't disappear overnight. I still had them. They felt a bit dented and bruised; I felt a hypocrite, but I was still the strong parent that I had always been. I still expected good manners, and taught the children a strong sense of right and wrong. I worked hard to ensure that the children maintained their family links with both sides of the family. Although I felt some anger and disappointment towards their father, I tried to keep this from them. I fought to ensure that they maintained their relationship with him, and kept in contact.

Life carries on, as it does. We all adjusted to life in a single-parent household. The children continued to develop. I began to wonder if the divorce was the awful thing that I had been waiting for, because it wasn't easy, but generally we got a good rhythm in the household.

I have always worked, choosing part-time hours and working a job share in order to look after my children. I left school at 16 and started work the following week in the head office of a regional building society, the Staffordshire. I took a maternity break when I had Nicholas and then decided to give up work altogether. However, after Anthony was born I decided to go back into financial services and took a part-time job at another building society, Birmingham Midshires. I started off in a small way by working Saturday mornings and covering holidays. Over the years as the children grew I gradually increased my hours until I was working a job share in the Internal Audit department. I really enjoyed my work and looked for opportunities to develop my career, eventually moving into project work. It was difficult trying to juggle everything; I had a strong feeling that I wanted to maintain a part-time contract so that I could enjoy the best of both worlds – work and being a mom. I only moved back into full-time employment through necessity after my divorce, but even then I waited until Krystie started full-time school. Following the divorce it was tough financially and I really struggled. On top of all the financial pressures I felt terribly guilty, and was driven to make sure that my children had all the emotional support that they needed. In the end, I was the one who got worn out, trying to be all things to all men.

While the boys grew, Krystie remained petite and dainty. Actually she seemed *too* small. She always seemed frail. My father summed it up once when he asked, 'Molvia, why doesn't Krystie seem to thrive?' Krystie did have a few problems that didn't seem right to me. She was referred to a paediatrician twice between the ages of 2 and 6. I had her referred because of odd symptoms such as tremors and shakes in her hands and legs. Another time because she used to panic if she thought that she wouldn't be able to get to a toilet quickly. It was like taking your granny out. Every day the same question: Where are we going, are we walking or are we in the car? If she thought that our trip involved a long stretch on the motorway, for example, she would get upset and worry that she would wet herself. None of it added up for me. She was the earliest of all of my children to toilet train. Within days of coming out of nappies, she was also dry at night. She has never had an accident. So none of this made sense. However, all the hospital tests proved to be clear. I started to think that I was neurotic, and that perhaps the divorce had affected her and that her anxiety was manifesting itself in these odd ways.

During this time I met the man who was to become my second husband, Mitchell. I met him when I was assigned to a new project team at work. We got on really well. I soon told him about my children, but he didn't meet them at that time. We 'dated' for several months before I eventually introduced him to them. They all got on really well. We decided to wait and see how our relationship developed, so he kept his flat and I lived with the children. We both felt that it was quite important for the children to be settled, and I wanted them to feel that they had time to get used to Mitchell. We all went out together on the weekends when they stayed home with me.

Mitchell used to say that he felt that Krystie wasn't walking properly. He compared her walking line to a crab; this was true, for example if you walked along the pavement in a straight line, Krystie would eventually walk into you. She didn't seem able to walk in a straight line. I explained that I had taken her to the hospital on several occasions but that they had assured me that she was fine. He thought that I should take her back to the doctor. I wasn't sure what to do. I began to worry that if I took her back to the doctors too often that someone would think that 'I' was ill! I had kept the memory of the police officers waiting to meet Anthony's ambulance a few years ago. I wasn't sure what the authorities would think about a single mom who appeared to have a neurotic fixation on her only daughter. I had read articles in the paper about children who had been taken away from parents because they were deemed to be unstable. I kept thinking that Andrew's death had made me paranoid. So, I stopped listening to that little voice in my head, my intuition; I ignored the things that I felt were strange and just carried on. Krystie was clumsy. She found it hard to balance and to run fast. She grew very slowly, and just seemed 'weak' to me, but I ignored my feelings. I still felt that something 'bad' was around the corner, but just pushed it to the back of my mind.

Even though I had been discharged from the hospital outpatient clinic a year or so earlier, I wasn't back to normal. Physical evidence of this were my periods, which were completely erratic, my weight, which was terrible to control, and my nerves, which were shaky. I never got back to be the person I was before I had Krystie. I had been fairly even, someone who never let anything get on top of me, with boundless energy. Our home was well organised even though I worked, and I always seemed to be on top of everything. Now, I got tired easily, and stressed about things. I found the fallout of divorce difficult. Forming another relationship contributed to the irritations that can occur around the subject of 'contact' and children.

My husband had a new partner; and I could understand that a woman might feel threatened by a man's ex-wife and her children. However, this insecurity can affect a man's choice to be consistent with his access arrangements. I could see that sometimes my ex-husband was in a situation where his apparent willingness to be co-operative with me caused pressure for him. This meant that as far as his partner was concerned the child access arrangements had to be inflexible for me. For example, if we agreed that the children would visit them every other weekend it had to be that way. I could not alter the arrangements, and there would be no contact in between. I had always explained to their father that he could visit his children in between times if he wanted to, or pick them up for an evening or telephone them.

Basically I wanted him to see as much as possible of them. I suppose that a third party can see this co-operation as evidence of an attachment or as a sign that the divorced couple may re-unite. Of course it's not about that, it's about maintaining strong links between the children and their absent parent. I believed that this was vitally important. The other problem that we had was the fact that arrangements on his side were altered at short notice. When I was single and on my own, this annoyed me (because the children were disappointed) but I didn't mind altering my plans. However, once I met Mitchell, it added a further complication. From his point of view, he looked forward to the small amount of time we had on our own. We usually planned to go out and meet friends, so unexpected changes upset long-standing arrangements. I could understand his frustration, after all he had been a bachelor who was free to come and go as he pleased. Not only did he have a woman to consider now, but also three children. I felt torn in two directions. I just wanted my ex and his partner to focus on the children and I wanted Mitchell not to get so wound up about cancelled arrangements. The most important thing for me was the children and a stable relationship with their father. If I had not cared about this, I do wonder what might have happened.

My ex-husband and his partner saw my trying to make alternative arrangements as my wanting to have a sense of power, which it wasn't at all. It was honestly about three children who I believed needed to stay in good contact with their father. I felt that whatever frustrations we shared, that they should maintain a good relationship with him. Looking back I can now see that my commitment to this added a mountain of pressure to my life, which all came to a head.

One weekend the children were due to be with their father on a Saturday evening and stay overnight. He called to say that his partner wasn't feeling too well so he would not be collecting them that weekend. I asked him what was wrong with her, but when he explained, it didn't sound like something that was really bad. I pointed out that generally parents had their children even if they were ill, and since it was only to be overnight and a few hours the next day I couldn't understand why they felt it was such a problem. We ended up arguing about it, and the call ended with him saying that he would not be collecting them. As often happened he also took the opportunity to remind me of everything he felt was wrong with me, and made out that I was being unreasonable. It was another upsetting incident. Then when I put the phone down, I had to tell the children that they would not be going away that afternoon, and tell them in a manner that was calm and rational without displaying my emotion. Of course they were disappointed. Next I had to contact Mitch and tell him that I wouldn't be able to make our plans that evening. He was really annoyed, and ended up by stating that I never ever seemed to put him first. I was trapped in the middle, and just felt that I was no good to anyone. About an hour later, their father called to say that he would collect the children after all, and so called round for them later on that afternoon; he was still annoyed with me and made that perfectly clear. When I called Mitchell to tell him that I could join him after all, he was still angry, and so that conversation also ended on a bad note. He did call round to see me, but we ended up arguing because he could not accept that I could not make my ex-husband stick to arrangements. He walked out in temper. What could I do? I had never really used babysitters, just members of my family. But everyone has lives to live and you can only ask people to do so much. I was also aware that three children were a lot for anybody. They did spend some time with grandparents, but I was a working mother and I needed and wanted to spend some quality time with them too. It was a delicate juggling act. When situations like that Saturday afternoon occurred I had to think what had happened in the preceding week, i.e. how often had the children been with their grandparents. If they had already spent a good amount of time with them I didn't like to just ring up my parents and expect them to change their plans yet again. It was all very difficult.

In the silence of that early Saturday evening I felt completely hopeless. I wasn't trying to dominate my ex-husband's relationship, I just wanted him to be consistent but also flexible on occasion, yet he always tried to make out that I was being completely selfish. When I thought about Mitchell, I felt that I was letting him down. I knew that he was really patient about the situation, but just needed him to understand that I wasn't in control of the arrangements. This was the key: Mitchell didn't like the fact that my ex had control. But then in the middle of all of this were the children; I was doing my absolute level best to keep them out of this. I wanted them to 'feel' good about their father. I didn't expect them to understand the undercurrents, and didn't want them to be aware of them. I just wanted all the adults in this to think about the children. I couldn't see the tension lifting; I felt that I was the source of all the trouble and that if I wasn't around everything would be calmer. I had reached breaking point and wanted everything to stop and be calm again. I think that over the years I had always been calm Molvia, the person who sorted things out, organised everything, listened to everyone, tried to help, and I just couldn't take anymore. I walked to the cupboard in the kitchen, and found my antidepressant tablets. I sat on the floor and took one after the other. I can't really remember how many I took; I know that it was quite a lot. I went and lay down on the sofa in the lounge and felt really peaceful. After about half an hour I started to feel unwell. Then I got scared. I started to think about the children. I realised that I was the one constant thing in their lives; I had brought them up well, and I was a good parent. I wondered what would happen if I wasn't around, and I started to panic. I didn't want to die. I telephoned Mitchell, feeling a mixture of stupid and scared, and he came round to take me to the hospital. The staff said that the tablets that I had taken were very dangerous and affected heart function; they pumped my stomach out, but said that I would have to be monitored because they could not be sure how much had got into my system. I was really frightened and so, so ashamed. Even as I write this I feel bitterly ashamed that people who know me will see this. But it did happen; it's part of my past. I had hit rock-bottom.

I stayed in hospital overnight, and was interviewed by a psychiatrist the following lunchtime. I found myself telling him about my childhood, all the traumas with Anthony, Krystie's birth and my divorce and the pressures that I now felt. He said that whilst I was experiencing a lot, I had to take time out for me, and not try to fix things for everyone. He said that he did not consider that I was a 'danger' or seriously mentally ill, just very depressed. He said that I had experienced a lot of stressful things, and that it seemed that I had always been the 'coper' in these situations, which meant that I had never really allowed myself to get over things properly. We talked about counselling, and he recommended that I talk to my doctor about arranging some sessions. They allowed me to go home.

Mitchell was shocked; he says now that he couldn't believe it. I was the last person that he would have considered would do something like that. My ex-husband was shocked too. My parents were so sorry. They asked me why I had not called them about the children. I tried to explain that it wasn't about the children, but more about being stuck in a con-tinuous battle situation. I was trying to be fair to everyone, but felt that I got very little co-operation back. I also said that I didn't want to burden them all the time. They said that I should always call them, and that they didn't mind my asking them to help with the children. My mother said that she thought that I always tried to do too much on my own, and that I shouldn't. She felt that she had contributed to that by everything that happened around the time of Andrew's death. I told her not to even think about that because it had happened a long time ago and wasn't worth dwelling on.

I did feel completely horrified at myself. I still do. I cannot believe that I had nearly abandoned my children who I love so much. It made me realise that I had to change. That I couldn't always be strong, and that I needed to take care of me. From that time on, things did ease. My ex-husband and his partner seemed to be more co-operative, and Mitchell became less stressed about it all. I made sure that anything important that Mitch and I wanted to do had completely separate child-care arrangements (i.e. was not dependent on their father). I also looked into alternative therapies for my hormone imbalance (that still existed), and found a practitioner who advised me on diet and supplements. I did arrange some counselling sessions through my GP. Everything started to look better. The whole experience made me realise that no matter how bad things get, you just have to face them. There is never a quick fix, or a way out, but over time things have a way of sorting themselves out. I also realised that I didn't have to be perfect, and that I didn't have to put everything right. The world wasn't going to stop if I took a step back. It was a valuable lesson, and one that has continued to serve me well.

One of the most difficult things I have ever had to do was sit down with my two boys and explain what I had done. They knew that I had been in hospital and wondered why; I thought that it was best to be honest. I explained that I had felt under pressure, and a little bit about the reason why. I also told them about why my nerves were weak (the hormone imbalance, and all the stressful things that had happened in the past) and how the feeling of being caught in the middle had just made me reach rock-bottom. I said that it was not about them, and explained that when I started to feel ill that I had been terrified that I was going to leave them alone. I told them that they must not look at me as a good example, and they must never ever think that what I had done was the solution, because it wasn't. They listened and asked questions; they said that I shouldn't worry about them and their dad, and that although they did like to see him regularly, they understood that he sometimes was just trying to keep the peace at home, and they therefore just enjoyed the time that they did have with him. They were so mature, and they said that they didn't think that I had done a very sensible thing (which I hadn't) and that they definitely wouldn't be copying me in the future. They were brilliant really, but I do not feel proud that we ever had to have that conversation, yet I am glad that I was honest with them, they deserved that. They also said that they were very happy with their life and that I didn't need to worry about everything so much, they were fine. Krystie was still very young; she was oblivious to everything. Thank goodness.

Despite everything that happened at this time, the children did maintain some contact with their father. I am not so naive to imagine that they do not have their own feelings about all of this, but they have become well-adjusted young people with a zest for life. They still have a relationship with their father, and neither of us resent time spent with the other. Children grow up, and over the years they began to make their own contact arrangements, which meant that I wasn't involved at all, and this made it easier for his new partner. I stopped feeling responsible for their relationship with their dad, as this was up to him. The truth is that children accept their parents, 'warts and all'.

When I think about that time, I wonder if some other factors contributed to my state of mind on that day. The first is that it happened when I was due for my period, and so I had PMT. PMT has caused me terrible problems over the years (obviously because of the hormone imbalance). After the birth of Krystie, when my hormones were disturbed, my monthly cycle was completely out of kilter. I had to take hormone replacement therapy for a time. In fact it's only been since the year 2001 that I have had a regular cycle. I only achieved this after years of experimenting with a blend of supplements. Once I managed to get my cycle sorted out, I noticed that my PMT became a much smaller problem. I had also had an operation under anaesthetic just a few weeks before the incident. I had a lump in my right breast that had to be removed. Fortunately it was not cancerous, but I had found the whole episode very worrying, and apparently anaesthetic can predispose you to depression. The other factor is the antidepressants that I was given. Due to my hormone imbalance I visited the doctor quite regularly. He was aware that my nerves were weak, and so I was given repeat prescriptions of these over the years. I would collect the prescription, and maybe take them for a few days or a couple of weeks, but then stop taking them because I didn't want to be addicted. I had gone through a period of taking them just prior to the suicide attempt. Later I came across articles in the press about Seroxat. These articles linked the drug to suicides in a number of people that had taken it. When I read the newspaper articles the name of the drug sounded familiar, so I cut one of the articles out of the paper and visited my doctor to ask him to go back to my records and check the name of the antidepressants that I had been taking. They were indeed Seroxat.

The greatest lesson of all from this episode was that I am human – not superhuman. I am not perfect and like most people I am flawed in some way.

Mitchell and I decided to get married the following year and set up home together. We had been together just over three years. I'm glad that we didn't rush things. The children felt secure with me, and needed time to get used to Mitchell. It was the same for him too. He had been a confirmed bachelor, so he needed time to adjust to the thought and the reality of taking on three children. When we got married Krystie was 7, Anthony 12 and Nicholas 14. We had a small family wedding, the children were involved and it was a lovely day.

Mitchell and I had agreed that I should start my own business just before we got married. It was something that I really wanted to do, because I wanted the independence. I drew on my experience of working in business re-engineering and start-ups to found a business consultancy. The business has given us some excellent opportunities, but has also afforded me the luxury of choice and flexibility when juggling work and family. Mitchell joined the business about a year after our wedding. The nature of our business has given us the ability to provide a comfortable home, a decent standing of living and a measure of financial security. We have been able to enjoy some precious family holidays together, which have given us some wonderful memories. It has also taught the children the value of hard work and the importance of pulling together.

We got married in April 1997, and in July of that year Mitchell's job transferred him out to South Carolina in the United States. I was pleased for him, but concerned because we had only just got married. However, I was able to secure work with his company, which meant that we could all join him in America. Actually Nicholas was just about to start his GCSE year at school, so he decided that he would prefer to stay in England. We made arrangements for him to stay with his grandparents, and Anthony and Krystie came with us. We moved out during the summer holidays, which meant that Nicholas could come with us for a holiday. We had a lovely apartment in a gated complex with two swimming pools and tennis courts. The children loved it. Nicholas flew home in time to start his new school term and Anthony and Krystie enrolled at the local schools. They had a great experience of 'American' school life. They caught the famous yellow school buses (what a great system!) and made friends quickly. Krystie was 7 at this time. When I look back at photographs now, I can see that she used to stand awkwardly and seemed very tiny. Nicholas flew out to join us for his October and Christmas holidays. We made the most of our time in America, visiting various places including Disneyworld in Florida, and generally we were very happy. But in 1998 I decided that I needed to return to England. I wasn't happy about the way that things were going with my job and I was missing Nicholas so I returned to the UK with Krystie in January of that year. I started a new freelance contract with Prudential and worked on the launch of Egg (the bank). Mitchell stayed in America with Anthony who would return to England in time to start the new term at the end of February. I found a house for us to rent and got Nicholas and Krystie settled before Anthony joined us just a few weeks later.

Mitchell decided to join the business and so he left America in April and joined the Prudential project to work on the bank launch too. I must have got pregnant almost as soon as he returned to England.

One night in 1998 I woke up from my sleep in a complete panic. I sat bolt upright in my bed. I was dripping with sweat and immediately started feeling at the side of my bed for a crib. I had the strongest feeling that I would find a baby. Then I realised that I had been dreaming. The dream came back to me. I had been lying in a hospital bed surrounded by doctors. I was looking at bright lights above me, and I had just had a little boy. It was a strange dream, because my previous experience of birth had been myself, my partner and two midwives. Still in a bit of a panic, I woke Mitch and explained the dream. I told him that I was pregnant and that I was going to have a boy. He was half asleep, but said 'You're having a nightmare, go back to sleep' (we laugh about this now). I did manage to go back to sleep, and put it all to the back of my mind.

About a month later I was feeling so tired. I had been working on a recruitment campaign up in Nottingham for two days and was completely exhausted. I decided to buy a pregnancy test. I did the test, and it was positive. My dream had been right. Even though the pregnancy was unplanned we were overjoyed. As a family we were all really pleased. Even my older boys (by now in their mid-teens) were really excited. I personally felt that a child would tie us all together, and so did Mitch. I spoke to my herbalist about the depression that I had suffered and he advised me to start taking some supplements when I reached 36 weeks that, he said, would really help my hormone balances. I really trusted him now, and so I wasn't worried. This time my pregnancy went really well. I had a little bit of morning sickness, and felt tired, but nothing like with my first three children. I was so glad not to experience that overwhelming 'ill' feeling that I had felt three times before. I did actually think about the fact that I had a new partner now, and therefore the genetic mix was different. I didn't dwell on it, but the thought did cross my mind.

At 30 weeks I woke up one morning to find I was bleeding. I called my mother-in-law to ask her to take the children to school for me. I then called my mother, and asked her to make her way over to my house later that day, so that she could be home when the children got back from school. My mother couldn't drive at that time so I was never able to call on her in an emergency if I needed someone to be with me quickly. She would always help, but was reliant on public transport. Anyway she agreed to come to our home later that day. I called Mitch who was already at work and asked him to leave and meet me at the hospital. I remember travelling in the ambulance thinking that maybe this was the 'bad' thing that I had been waiting for.

Once I arrived they carried out some tests and scanned me. They explained that I had placenta praevia, and that the placenta was lying below my baby. They said that this was life-threatening for both the baby and me. I was put on immediate bed rest. It became clear that I would not be allowed to go back home until the baby was born. They also explained that placenta praevia could result in a massive haemorrhage, and if this happened and they could not stop the bleeding that it could prove fatal. Both Mitch and I were shattered. I had three children at home and Krystie was only 8. I could not imagine spending the next ten weeks flat on my back in hospital. I didn't want to think that the baby, Mitchell's first baby, and I might die. I had no choice I had to stay in hospital. The boys were really helpful, and my mother moved in to look after everybody. At 34 weeks I haemorrhaged again. I spent the best part of a day in a delivery suite trickling blood into a bucket very, very slowly. I started bleeding at about 5 o'clock in the morning and stopped at about 3 o'clock in the afternoon. Fortunately it was a very light bleed (placenta praevia can cause the placenta to tear away from the womb, which can result in a woman bleeding to death in a matter of minutes). I was scared, but I got through it. The following day my obstetrician met with me, and explained that I really couldn't afford to have another bleed. He said that he didn't really want to deliver the baby yet because I was only 34 weeks, and he felt that it could be dangerous for the baby. Instead he talked me through a plan of action, which was that he would put me on 'very strict' bed rest (allowed up for the toilet and meals only), and start injections that would strengthen the baby's lungs. He said that he would scan me once a week to check the baby and was planning to deliver it by a Caesarean section at exactly 36 weeks. So basically I just had to get through the next fortnight.

On Thursday, 27 November 1998 I was taken to the delivery suite; everything was prepared and they administered the spinal block for the Caesarean. After about ten minutes I started to feel unwell; I was not reacting well to the spinal block, my heart was doing strange things, I was drifting in and out of consciousness. Mitchell has told me that it was like a mad house; the anaesthetist was injecting me in my arm every few minutes. Mitch remembers watching him give me at least twelve injections; the team were shouting at each other, people were rushing around. As for me I was back in my dream, the lights above me were appearing and disappearing depending on whether I was conscious or not. I was indeed surrounded by doctors in masks, and I did deliver a little boy; we called him Harrison.

He screamed before he was pulled out of my womb. As soon as the doctor touched him he cried. The doctor said that a baby hadn't done that before. As soon as I heard him, I turned to Mitch and said that he sounded funny but he was handed to me, and everyone thought that he was fine. He weighed 7lb 4 oz, so considering that he was four weeks early was a very healthy weight; in fact he was the heaviest baby that I had had! Despite this I really didn't like the noise he was making. I called the nurse, she checked him, held him for a while, and assured me that he was fine. We were in the ante-room for about ten minutes and all this time he kept making his strange little sound. I really didn't like it; it was a completely different sound to my other children, but no one else seemed bothered. We were all taken back to my room. I held him and tried to feed him, but he wouldn't latch on, he was stretching his neck back. His fingertips, toes and lips seemed tinged with blue. I kept trying to settle him but an hour later he was no better. We called a midwife and asked for a paediatric nurse to come and see him. She came, and agreed that perhaps he needed a 'little bit' of oxygen. She took him away and suggested I take a little rest. I felt happy that Harrison was being looked after, so I went to sleep.

Mitchell took my mother home and we agreed that when he got back we would fetch Harrison together. Mitchell got back and his sister arrived at the same time. I sat in a wheelchair (because I had only had my Caesarean a few hours previously) and we all went to fetch Harrison, but when we got to the neonatal unit we were not allowed into the room where Harrison was. Three doctors were huddled around an incubator, and a nurse shouted that the doctors were operating on a little baby. She literally slammed the door in our faces so that we couldn't enter the room. I looked at the name board and cot positions information hanging in the corridor and realised quickly that they were working on Harrison. I shouted back at the nurse that the baby they were operating on (her words) was my baby, so what the hell was going on, since I had been told that my baby just needed a little oxygen. The fear in my mind was like a vice. I kept thinking that this was the bad thing that I had been waiting for all my life. I looked at Mitchell and felt so sad that this was his baby, his first baby. The nurse shouted that he had 'grotty lungs', and that they were really bad. She ushered us into a room. Mitchell and his sister were in silent shock; I was 'feisty' Molvia. How dare this woman shout at me, about our baby; this nurse, one of those people who had spent over an hour telling me that my baby was fine, when I kept saying that he wasn't? I demanded that she tell me immediately what was going on, and shouted, 'Get me a doctor now!!!' The doctor came; she explained that Harrison had respiratory distress syndrome, and that the best odds they could give him were 50/50. Once she had explained everything, and once I had asked every question in my mind, I slumped back into my wheelchair and cried.

We spent the next five days in limbo. He was such a big baby compared to all the other tiny babies in their incubators, but he was just as poorly. He was big because I had had high sugar when I carried him (gestational diabetes), which had not been picked up. It meant that he was a big baby with immature lungs. It was terrible watching him, not knowing if he was going to make it or not. I kept thinking that this must definitely be the bad thing that I had been expecting. I just couldn't believe that this was Mitchell's first experience of childbirth, and I really didn't want his child to die. On day five Harrison suddenly turned the corner and never looked back. On day seven he was allowed down on to the ward with me. We went home a few days later. Unfortunately, he developed severe jaundice on his second day at home so we were rushed back into hospital. He spent four days under lights. His bilirubin levels were dangerously high, just below the point where doctors advise a complete blood exchange. However, once again he battled, turned the corner and got well.

I remember the night before we were due to return home sitting on my bed holding him. It was about eleven o'clock at night, dark and quiet. I looked down at this little miracle again. I felt so happy. I thought about all my babies. I was such a lucky woman. I thought about my divorce, and meeting Mitchell. I thought about the fact that he had taken on my three children, and had seemed to adapt really well. Harrison was the icing on the cake. Tears filled my eyes, and then I went stone cold. I just had this feeling that everything was too good to be true. I had this overwhelming feeling that something was definitely going to go wrong. I felt really scared; I shivered physically, and hugged Harrison to me tightly. I told myself not to be silly, I blamed 'baby blues' and once again pushed that nagging feeling to the back of my mind. Looking back I don't think it was baby blues, it was definitely intuition.

A swimming lesson 3

Once I got back home, things settled back into a routine. I had been away from home for about ten weeks altogether. My older children had visited me during that time, but time away makes you see things differently.

It was just after Christmas, and the health visitor had called to check on Harrison. I knew her really well. She had been my health visitor with my older children, so we chatted easily. I explained that I was not really worried about the baby. Despite his initial problems he was doing really well. He was feeding and sleeping, responding to me readily and as far as I was concerned was a complcte delight. On the other hand what I did want her to do was look at Krystie.

I had been in hospital for a long time. Now that I was back home, I had noticed how clumsy Krystie 'really' was. She stumbled all the time. We had double doors into our lounge, and an archway into our dining room, but whenever she passed through these doorways she seemed to bounce off both sides. As she walked, she seemed to walk with a lurch. Over the days since my return I was convinced that something was wrong. I sat next to the health visitor and together we watched Krystie. I asked her to walk up and down the lounge and through the doors into the hallway. The health visitor agreed that she was clumsy. She also remarked that Krystie had always been small and petite (to illustrate, Krystie was nearly 9, and wore age 5 to 6 clothes, sometimes age 7), but she ended her remarks by saying perhaps I shouldn't worry. She didn't seem too concerned, but she did say that if I was really worried that I should take her back to the doctor. I didn't take her.

I have sat and wondered about this so many times. I did believe, and had always believed, that something wasn't quite right. I didn't like the way Krystie walked. Just before Harrison was born my father had strongly advised me to take her to the doctor, because in his opinion he felt that she was too small and sort of weak. I think looking back that I was scared. Scared that he and I were right, and scared of the unknown.

I coped with the new baby really well. I took the supplements that my herbalist had recommended, and they really did the trick because I just didn't seem to suffer with post-natal depression at all.

I decided that Krystie should have swimming lessons. She seemed to struggle with physical activities, and still could not swim. So I enrolled her at a swimming club and turned up for her first lesson. It was bustling with activity. A mix of parents and children, moisture from the pool and the smell of chlorine. I had Harrison in his baby seat, and got Krystie changed. I watched her for ten minutes, and then dashed off to squeeze a visit to the post office in. I did my jobs, and rushed back just in time to get her dried and changed. As I walked in through the door, the manager of the swimming club Gina approached me. 'Are you Krystie's mom?' she asked. 'Yes,' I replied. She looked at me and grabbed my arm, and said 'What is wrong with your daughter?' She was talking quickly and a bit excitedly, there was an urgency in her voice; she caught me off guard. 'Nothing, there's nothing wrong with her,' I answered. She looked at me, and realised that she had startled me. 'It's OK,' she said, 'but when we got Krystie out of the pool, she was shaking so much that she couldn't stand properly. I just thought that it wasn't right that's all.' I nodded at her and explained that this did happen sometimes. I also explained that I had taken her to the hospital about it in the past and they had said that she was fine. At this, Gina got really insistent. She grabbed my arm again, and said, 'No, you must take her back, do you hear me? I have seen so many children over the years and this isn't right.' In that moment, it was as if the world disappeared, all I could see were Gina's lips moving up and down as if in slow motion. Nothing else existed, her voice seemed to be slow and deep and loud. In that instant all that was in focus were her words, and the realisation that I *had* been right all along. I knew I would take her back to the doctor, and this time I wouldn't stop until they found out what was wrong. The world came back, and Gina was demanding that I took her to casualty that evening. I reassured her that I would take her to the doctor not this evening but first thing on Monday (this was a Friday evening). I told her that it wouldn't be right to take her to casualty tonight, but I would go through the proper channels and would definitely get it sorted out. As soon as we got home I telephoned the doctor's surgery and got an appointment for the following Monday morning.

Monday came quickly and we visited the doctor. I explained our history, and my recent worries. I told him about the swimming lesson, and he asked Krystie to walk. As she walked and we both watched her, it was apparent that something was wrong. He agreed to refer her immediately. He explained that he would send a letter off that day, and that we would get an appointment through the post. I asked him if he knew how long it would take. He said that he wasn't sure. It was the end of February now, and although we didn't realise it, we had just started the waiting game.

Krystie

Ah, the infamous swimming lesson. I always did loathe swimming; too cold for my liking. Anyway, yes, I do remember that day well. I was 9 and mom had booked swimming lessons for me, due to the fact that I just wasn't picking it up on my own, or with her help. Nik and Ant always joked that they should do to me what they did with my granddad. Chuck me in a river and hope I float! Whether or not that actually happened is anyone's guess. It got to the end of the lesson and the whistle blew. I got out of the pool; not surprisingly, I was cold, and when I was cold I shook quite a lot. One of the instructors helped me to the showers. I don't really remember what happened in between that, but I did have a shower and then . . . I think mom was pulled over by the swimming instructor who helped me out of the pool. She began talking to mom about me. I can just about remember picking up on the fact that she thought something was wrong with me, something serious.

'I was just cold and a bit tired,' I assured them both, again and again. I was getting worried about where the conversation was headed. Then again, as I said, I knew something was wrong, and I knew it'd all have to come out in the end.

The waiting game

4

I find it really hard to wait. Once I have made a decision, I just like to get on with it. I am the sort of person who likes to know the facts and details; once I understand everything I can cope. However, I was not in control of this – we were dependant on the National Health Service. Thankfully her appointment came through fairly quickly, I think that it was around the end of March, 1999.

On the day of the appointment they did all the usual things, height, weight and details of her medical history. Then they started to do the other examinations. Krystie lay on a couch. Dr Anderson (Consultant Obstetric Paediatrician) examined her chest and joints. Then she tested her reflexes, only they didn't work. The doctor tapped her knees with the little rubber hammer and they didn't move. Next she asked Krystie to touch her own nose with her index finger and then move the finger in a straight line to touch the doctor's finger that she was holding up. Krystie couldn't do it. Well, she could, but her finger took a major detour before it made contact with the doctor's finger. You should be able to do it in a smooth movement. Krystie couldn't. I watched and felt sick. Then Krystie had to walk and hop. She was so off balance; I knew that they wouldn't tell me that she was 'OK' this time. Krystie had blood taken for some tests. She was amazing, she didn't cry, she just sat there while they filled several little bottles of blood. The doctor explained that she needed to begin a range of investigations on Krystie starting with an MRI scan. It was clear that we were not going to get answers overnight; we would just have to be patient.

Krystie

Hmmm, meeting Dr Anderson, well that was fun. I had many tests done that day, none quite as unforgettable as the 'touch your nose, touch my finger' test in which I basically had to, well, touch my nose, then touch Dr Anderson's finger, alternating between the two. I was okay at first then, as I was asked to increase my speed, I began to make mistakes, poking my eye, missing her finger. It was awful, funny, but awful. At first the tests were fun and I felt special. I always did like being the centre of attention, plus at that stage I had no idea what the tests were for either. Soon, however, I was bored, and though they kept me occupied I couldn't help but think what the hell were all these pointless tasks gonna prove? Still I managed to keep myself and people around me entertained with my very — dare I say it — dry, sarcastic sense of humour. Finally, after what seemed like weeks of waiting — though in actual fact it was merely a day — and of endless blood-taking and (what I can only describe as) fitness tests, I was released, and then began the wait.

A phrase that the doctor used stuck in my mind; she said that Krystie had an 'ataxic' walk. I remembered this so that I could look it up. Once we got home, I looked up the word ataxia, and read what I could. It wasn't very helpful; it suggested that Krystie could have a brain tumour or a genetic illness. I remember talking to my mother and saying, 'Well it can't be the genetic illness, because we haven't got anything wrong in our family have we?' She agreed that everyone in our family seemed fine. I wasn't overly distressed about the prospect of a tumour. Only a few months earlier, one of my work colleagues had watched her sister cope with a brain tumour. I remembered that they had managed to take it away and now she was fine. My cleaner's husband had also survived a brain tumour, and was perfectly happy and healthy. The scan couldn't come quickly enough for me, I just wanted to know! Krystie didn't really ask very much. She was quite unconcerned and didn't complain about anything. She was her usual happy little self.

Two weeks later we took Krystie to Birmingham for an MRI scan. Again she was just so brave. She seemed so small climbing on to the big

MRI scanning table. The operator explained that she would need to lie completely still. Krystie joked that she was quite jerky but would try her best. The machine moved her tiny little body into the tunnel. I would have felt so claustrophobic, but she didn't moan at all. She lay there for twenty minutes while the machine made it's clunky noisy sounds as it took pictures of her brain. I was so relieved when it was all over, and very proud of her.

Krystie

The MRI scan, yes I remember that, how very exciting it was at the time. Back then I didn't really understand what it was all about so I wasn't scared about all these tests. Safe in the naive belief that only old people died. Now that I look back I realise just how young I was, and how stupid some of the things that I thought really were, but maybe, just maybe it was better that way. Fear could've destroyed me, destroyed who I was, who I am today; yes I was definitely better off.

Anyway, back to the MRI. Well the machine itself was a large doughnut shape, constantly making an annoying whirring sound. There was a large flat table protruding from the hole in the middle much like a tongue, which I was expected to lie on for half an hour — how uncomfortable! As the table began sliding into the machine I couldn't help but compare the scene to a James Bond film. Inside it was loud, and getting louder. It's hazy as to what really happened inside but I can remember being told to turn my head and such, and flippin' heck, did I have a headache, and that was it until the end really.

I sent Krystie out to Mitchell, and I hung back to wait for the radiographer. When she came out of her little room, I approached her and said, 'I know that you are not supposed to tell me anything, but please can you tell me, did you see anything unusual in her brain?' She looked at me as if she didn't know what to say. I looked back at her and said, 'I know that this is awkward for you, but believe me I want you to tell me that she has a brain tumour, because you can treat tumours, people have them taken away, but if she hasn't got a tumour, then she has something terrible, and I need to know, she's my daughter.' I didn't say it in an emotional fashion, just in a calm level manner. She studied my face and said, 'I didn't see any evidence of a tumour.' I thanked her and went back to Mitchell and Krystie.

We drove back to Wolverhampton. As Mitchell drove us home I was thinking that it was very strange that you could feel sad that your daughter didn't have a brain tumour. But I did. I just had this strong feeling that a tumour could probably be treated. On the other hand, I knew that a genetic illness could not. I knew that a genetic illness would be terrible. Once we got home I made sure everyone was all right and then went up to the main Wolverhampton library. I used the reference section to look at the medical textbooks. I pulled book after book off the shelves. I looked up the one root word that I had 'ataxia'. Every book kept bringing me back to genetic illnesses. One caught my eye, it was an illness called Friedreich's Ataxia (FA). I made a note of the name and went back home. Once home I logged on to the Internet and searched for information on this strange illness. What I read was like a slow dawn; the realisation crept over me. All the symptoms fitted Krystie. I logged on to an American information site where parents had registered their own personal experiences. A couple of the stories could have been ours. Even down to the strange fixation on the toilet, which, it turns out, is driven by the urgent need to pass water (not every sufferer experiences this, but some do). I stayed on the Internet into the early hours of the morning. I read anything and everything that I could find on the subject. After just a few hours I knew that my Krystie had Friedreich's Ataxia. I just knew. I also found out that I had to be a carrier of the faulty gene. I felt terrible, I felt like I had shot a bullet into my child. I felt like a murderer.

Friedreich's Ataxia is passed on to a child by two parents who each carry a faulty copy of gene number 9. This meant that Krystie's father and I carried the same faulty gene. Every human being carries pairs of genes. A developing foetus takes a copy of each gene from its father and mother to make its own new pair of genes. Krystie had acquired her father's faulty copy and mine. This meant that her number 9 gene had two faulty copies. Her father and I obviously only had one faulty copy each so we are only carriers of the illness, but because she had taken two faulty copies she had the illness and would display it. She had been unlucky.

A few days later I telephoned Dr Anderson's secretary, I asked her to pass a message on to the doctor for me. 'Could you please ask Doctor Anderson to look at Friedreich's Ataxia, because I have been doing some research, and I think that she might have this illness?' The secretary said that she would pass the message on for me. Dr Anderson telephoned me a few days later. She said that she couldn't say for sure what was wrong with Krystie, because she had to carry out a series of tests. Those tests would include the blood tests. Whilst she couldn't say yes or no to Friedreich's Ataxia, what she could say was that Krystie's illness was going to be something unusual and obscure. However, just a couple of weeks later, so I guess that it was early April, we received an appointment letter requesting that we meet Dr Anderson and a genetic specialist at the hospital. Krystie and I attended the appointment. Dr Anderson introduced us to the specialist. She explained Krystie's illness and together they repeated the reflex and index finger tests. Krystie walked up and down, and they also examined Krystie's hands (they hadn't done this before) and then Dr Anderson turned to me and said, tell the doctor what you asked me. I explained that I had been doing research, and that because of the various symptoms that I had read about, and because of the similar case histories that I had studied, I was wondering if Krystie had Friedreich's Ataxia. He looked at me, and said that he thought that it was highly likely that Krystie did have Friedreich's Ataxia, however they would not be in a position to give me a definitive answer until the blood results came through.

I didn't feel upset, or tearful. I was dealing in facts now and felt more comfortable. For the first time in my life that feeling of impending doom had gone. This was what I had been waiting for. This was the challenge that our family had to face. I had read the Internet; I knew that this illness was going to be terrible, but that horrible waiting had finished. I didn't quite appreciate that this would be replaced by the feeling of a continuous battle; that realisation would come later. We left the hospital and went home to wait for the blood test results. But I knew, I really did, I knew that Krystie had Friedreich's Ataxia.

Krystie

You know, it's hard to remember how I felt before we officially found out I had Friedreich's Ataxia; though I always had the feeling that there was something not quite right with me, ignoring the fact that I've always been slightly mental! I think the first time that I felt something wasn't right was when I was 5 or 6. We were at the assembly (convention for Jehovah's Witnesses). During the prayer I closed my eyes – as normal – but when I tried to stand without holding on to something I felt myself begin to wobble. I didn't feel at all stable. 'Strange' I thought opening my eyes, wondering what on earth could be the matter with me. I closed them once again. This time, however, I simply fell forwards. It didn't help that the convention was being held at the Wolverhampton football ground because I nearly toppled over the seat in front of me!

It was then, right then, that I knew something was wrong. Just a few weeks before I'd been able to stand perfectly well with no support at all. 'So why,' I wondered, 'couldn't I do it now?' From then on I started noticing things about me. Subtle things that only I or a close member of my family could notice. For example, I couldn't rollerblade – but then some people found it difficult at first. I was a slow runner – but so was my mom. I found it impossible to balance when at the ice rink – but so did a lot of people. These types of things and a few more, brushed aside each time they entered my mind, but always bothering me.

Later that day we sat down on the sofa to have a drink and have a chat about the hospital appointment. I had decided that we had to be honest with Krystie. I didn't feel that it was fair to hide anything from her. I had to balance this with the knowledge that she was only 9 (she had just had her birthday in March), and just a child. However, she knew that she didn't feel 'right' (her words). She knew that she was having tests to try and find out what was wrong with her. She had heard the name of a strange illness called Friedreich's Ataxia and she knew that this illness affected people's ability to walk. However, now she turned to me and asked, 'Mom, you know that doctor today, well he was checking my hands, why was he doing that?' I looked at her and asked, 'Why do you think he was doing that?' She hesitated and then said, 'Well I know that Friedreich's Ataxia affects your legs, but does it affect your hands too?' Her face looked so concerned, and I felt a lump in my throat, as I answered, 'Yes it does.' She looked horrified as she said, 'But I want to be an artist, how can I be an artist if my hands won't work. I won't be able to paint; I don't mind my legs so much but I do mind my hands.' Up until that point I had been fairly strong around Krystie. She knew that I was worried, and she knew that I was doing everything that I could to help find out what was wrong with her but she hadn't seen me cry. Now I did. I couldn't help it. Krystie loved her art, and she had wanted to be an artist since the age of 5. She was talented and loved to paint and draw. Her brothers used to tease her that artists never got rich until they died, but she didn't care, that is what she wanted to do. I knew how much this meant to her. I hugged her, and we sat and cried together. Looking back I think that it was good that she saw me cry, because it meant that she knew that you could have both sad and strong times. She needed to know that she could cry if she wanted to. After a few minutes I talked to her about the fact that art can be expressed in so many different ways. We talked about Van Gogh and the Impressionists. I said that she might end up on a stage one day, wheeling her chair through paint and creating great works of art in front of audiences of enthralled people! We both laughed and after a few moments, in true Krystie fashion, she looked at me and said, 'That's all very well mom, but I don't really like Impressionism, what I like is still life which requires exact lines and precision, so maybe I'll have to find something else to do.' I couldn't help but smile at her, but I also felt sad that already her dreams were being altered. I knew that this was only the start.

I explained to a few members of the family what the specialist had said, but we couldn't really tell many people because we had to have the definite blood results. We just had to wait.

One August Thursday evening, it was around seven o'clock, the telephone rang. I went to answer it. 'Hello, Mrs Maddox, this is Dr Anderson.' 'Hello,' I replied. She went on, 'We have had the results of the blood tests, and I am sorry to tell you that Krystie does have Friedreich's Ataxia, I'm very sorry.' 'That's OK,' I said, 'I knew. It's been like waiting for a bus, we just didn't know when it was coming.' 'I know, I know,' she answered. We exchanged a few more words; she explained that an appointment was being sent out to us, so that we could go in to talk to her. We said goodbye and I put the phone down. I remember thinking how nice it was that she had telephoned me in person, and that she was a lovely lady. I thought about the time of the evening, and how hard she worked. I went back to my usual evening tidy-up chores. Everything was oddly normal really. I remembered the doctor's explanation about the 'bad genetic mix' and thought about how sick I was when I carried my first three children. I had dismissed his comment, but look now: he might have been right. It's funny what you remember and think about when you are under stress. I felt that I should be screaming or crying; I wondered how I would tell Krystie that we actually knew for sure now. I felt strangely detached. I thought about everything that I had ever read about the illness and I could have just died realising what was to come. But even so I also felt a very strange sense of calm.

Explaining 'degenerative' to a child

5

How do you tell someone who has their whole life in front of them? How do you explain the extent of an illness, without destroying a child's 'zest' for life?

I went to find Krystie. I told her that Dr Anderson had telephoned me to tell me that the blood test results confirmed that she did have Friedreich's Ataxia. Krystie said that we had thought it was that and then added, 'Oh well that's that then – at least we know.' She asked me what would happen next, and I explained that we would be visiting Dr Anderson to talk about everything. I also told her that I would be looking into any alternative therapies that might be useful. She didn't agree that there would be any point in doing that. I gave her a hug and told her that she should try not to worry. She had various questions. She wanted to know when she would need a wheelchair, and what would happen. I could only tell her that no one really knew. She appeared to be taking the news well, and didn't seem overly upset. I guess that she was facing the unknown.

On top of this I had other children. I had to face the fact that my older sons could have the same illness as Krystie. I knew from my research that Friedreich's Ataxia has a common set of multiple symptoms, but no two people display them in the same way. I also knew that people could develop the symptoms at different ages. Some people started to display the symptoms early on in life, other people managed to get through their teens before the illness attacked. My sons were only young: Nicholas was 16 and Anthony 14. I wasn't so concerned about Harrison. He had a different father to my other children; I felt that it was highly unlikely that I would have been so unlucky to pick a second husband with the same faulty gene. Harrison could of course carry the gene, because he might have picked up a copy of my faulty number 9 gene, but I didn't expect him to actually have the illness.

All of this was very difficult for my boys. Just the same as every other family, they were and still are very different to each other. Nicholas was very calm and level-headed; he was a sensitive boy, very caring. Anthony on the other hand was gregarious, and hot-tempered; he was loving too – just different to Nicholas. I sat them down to talk to them about the results. I printed off information about Friedreich's Ataxia, and answered their questions. I explained that they would need to have blood tests to find out if they shared the same illness as Krystie. Nicholas said that he knew that he didn't have the illness, but that of course he would have the test. Anthony said that he didn't understand why he should have to be tested. He was quite upset. He said that he didn't want to know if he had the illness, and that I was wrong to expect him to be tested. I explained that I felt strongly that they should both know as quickly as possible. I felt that if they did share the condition, that we needed to look at all the alternative therapies that we could find, to help slow down the illness if at all possible. (This is what I had decided to do for Krystie.)

On the day of the test, we set off to the surgery. Anthony was like a cat on hot bricks, whilst Nicholas was calm. Anthony refused to get out of the car. I had to be really firm and tell him that I would drag him in there if necessary. I shouted at him, and asked him if he thought that I was enjoying this. I asked him to show some maturity and take the test. Nicholas spoke very calmly to him, and we walked into the surgery together. Anthony couldn't keep still. He got up, paced up and down, looked like he was going to burst into tears, and kept giving me angry looks. I felt so bad for him, and questioned myself inside, but I just had to make him do this. The receptionist called us through, and we all walked into the doctor's room. Anthony turned tail for the door, and I said, 'Anthony come and sit down.' I explained that he was finding this daunting, which of course brought out his teenage bravado, 'I'm fine,' he said defiantly and sat down. The doctor spoke to us about the test, and made sure that the boys understood its significance. Nicholas had his blood taken and was very calm. When it was Anthony's turn, he said, 'I can't believe you're making me do this mom.' He looked ready to

43

thump someone, and moaned when the needle went in. He said that it was hurting, and he was really tense. He was so glad when it was all over, and then just wanted to get out of the room as quickly as possible. We had to wait six weeks for the results.

The results came back. Once again we visited the surgery to collect them. Nicholas carried the faulty gene; he didn't have the illness but carried the gene. Anthony said 'I don't want to know'; he was really uncomfortable and angry with me. However, Anthony's results were the same as Nicholas's, and he only carried the faulty gene. We drove home. When we got home I tried to talk to the boys. Anthony was really upset, very emotional: 'Mom I feel such a baby. Krystie is so brave and strong, but I couldn't cope mom; if I had the illness, I would kill myself. I don't want her to have the illness but it's a good job that it's her and not me, and how bad is it for me to say that? I'm a coward, I am, but I wouldn't cope if I couldn't play my football and do my sports.' I hugged him, and told him not to be ashamed, I said that it was fine to be scared, and I also told him that he probably would cope if it were him. I told him that he wasn't a coward, and that he was normal. Nicholas got upset too. He said that he knew that he wouldn't have the illness; he just knew that he was going to be fine. But his eyes filled with tears when he said, 'But mom I wish it was me. She's just a little girl, it isn't fair. I wish I could have it instead of her.' He had a hug too. Two different reactions; two different people; both suffering each in their own way. Both perfectly valid; I didn't think one son was better than the other, I just thought that they were my boys. I was aware that the teenage years are stressful enough and made a mental note to talk to each of them on a one-to-one basis from time to time just to make sure that they could share their feelings if they wanted to.

I thought about the families that had two, three and four children with the illness. Some parents had all of their children diagnosed with it. My heart went out to them. There are no words.

Back to Krystie. I printed some information off the Internet and gave it to her so that she could read it. She asked me questions and I answered them as honestly as I could. I tried to explain things simply, and give positive explanations. One day she asked me if she was going to die. I looked at her and replied that we were *all* going to die. 'No mom,' she said. 'Will I get to grow up?' I took a breath, and said that I didn't know for sure. I put an arm around her and explained that Friedreich's Ataxia is different in every single person who has it. Some people die when they are young, other people grow older. I told her that we were going to try and find out as much as we could about the illness, and that we would try and find out about things that are called alternative therapies. I explained that we didn't know if they would help her, but that we would try. I also talked to her about the fact that none of us know what is going to happen to us. I remember saying that today some people will have said goodbye to their families, and then crashed their car never to return home. Some people will catch horrible viruses like meningitis today, and be dead by next week. I said that I didn't want to scare her, but she needed to realise that none of us can guarantee anything. Lots of people think they are perfectly healthy and have terrible accidents, and their lives are altered forever. So what she needed to do was just be glad for each and every day on its own. I also said that lots of people are perfectly healthy and yet they are so depressed and sad that they never leave their homes, never talk to other people but live alone, trapped in a world where they didn't do anything. On the other hand, some people who had severe disabilities or massive challenges just got on with life and enjoyed it. She looked at me and said, 'Yes, like that Professor Stephen Hawking. He has written that fantastic book hasn't he, and talks through that funny machine, he goes on telly and everything. If he can do it I can.' I told her that she was exactly right. I told her that of course it was sad that she had this illness, and that it would create challenges for us, but I said that there are always people worse off than we are, always. It was really up to her to be happy; if she set her mind to it, she could be. She smiled at me, and said 'I know mom, I know, at least I've got my family around me.'

We went along to see Dr Anderson. She talked to us about the illness. She explained that she couldn't offer us a cure, but what they would do was monitor its progression, treat individual symptoms as they occurred (if they could) and simply manage the illness. After a while she turned to Krystie and said, 'Do you have any questions?' Krystie looked at her and said, 'Just one. Has my mom told me everything about this illness, because I don't want people to hide anything from me? Even if it's bad, I want to know about it, because this is happening to me and it's my body.' We were all a little taken aback. The doctor smiled and said, 'I think your mom has told you everything Krystie, and if you have questions just ask her.' I knew then that I had been right to be as honest as I could with her.

I contacted the support organisation for Friedreich's Ataxia, called Ataxia UK. I spoke to them about Krystie, and they were really positive. It was good to talk to people who knew the implications of the illness. They were realistic, but also told me about other young people who were able to get on with their lives. I decided to join the organisation, which meant that we receive regular newsletters that are encouraging, and give details of the research that is carried out. They hold an annual AGM and dinner dance, which enables you to meet families in similar circumstances if you want to.

Over the years, as the illness progresses, Krystie has had questions and queries along the way. I took the decision to be honest with her, and at times that has been difficult. Sometimes the facts have been stark and cruel. This has caused me to think long and hard about the way that I explain things to her. I have tried to take the sting out of the information, and balance it with practical ways that we can manage that particular aspect of the illness. I have never forgotten Krystie's explanation about the fact that she 'knew what was happening to her body before anyone else did'. That makes sense to me; like when you get the tickle in your throat before you get the sore throat, or the tingle on your lip before a cold sore develops. We can think that we are helping our children by hiding the facts, but I think that this can be confusing. You might tell them one thing, but their body feels something completely different and they can't make sense of it. I believe that *this* confusion can cause additional stress and worry. Children are more astute than we give them credit for, even at a young age; I have always believed that they should be treated with respect; for me being honest is part of that respect.

Friedreich's Ataxia is a degenerative illness. This means that there is no cure, and that gradually over time the symptoms increase and get worse. It is an illness that affects the neurological pathways around the body. So messages leave the brain, but the nerve pathways that they use break down, messages cannot travel smoothly or even not at all. Over time the legs are affected so that the sufferer develops the 'ataxic' walk which means that people walk as if they are drunk. Eventually they cannot walk at all. It also affects the hands and arms, so that it is difficult to hold things without shaking. This affects practical day-to-day things like writing, eating and drinking. The neck can develop a tremor. It can also affect hearing and speech. Other organs can be affected so the heart can become enlarged, bladder control can become weak. The spine can curve (scoliosis), and the feet become deformed. A person's ability to swallow smoothly can be affected so that they choke easily on food. It is common for sufferers to develop diabetes. It is a terrible illness, where any one of these multiple symptoms (or a combination of them) can ultimately shorten the life of the sufferer. However, no two people are the same; the illness develops at different rates. Some people manage the illness into their fifties and beyond, other people have a shortened life.

Krystie started to display the symptoms of this illness when she was about 6. Medical opinion is that a sufferer will usually be a full-time wheelchair user within five years of diagnosis. Krystie became a full-time wheelchair user at 13.

I have often wished that she could have had her teenage years without the diagnosis. I have met other sufferers who were not diagnosed until they were 17 or 18. It would have been nice for Krystie to have experienced her school years without this illness. I have been told that she has an aggressive form of Friedreich's Ataxia, which means that she has multiple symptoms that have attacked her quite quickly.

None of it has been a shock to me, because I researched so much at the beginning. I have always been aware of the impact and I also understand how it may progress further. I prefer to be this way. I have spoken with other mothers who do not want to know what is going to happen. People are very different, you cannot judge until you have lived through the experience. Every parent does what they feel is right and best at the time. As I write about all of this I know that it seems like I was fairly calm and level-headed about everything, but in reality that's not how I always felt. If I brooded over the future and if I ever pictured Krystie far ahead in the future badly affected by the illness, possibly blind and deaf with limbs that shook badly and a throat that choked as she tried to swallow, I felt overwhelmed. I didn't want to see her like that, knowing that her brain would still be completely fine. That is to say that she would know exactly what was happening to her. Krystie is such a vibrant character; she is so full of life and so completely knows what she wants that I cannot imagine it. In those early days when I allowed myself to feel morose about everything I considered the possibility of perhaps giving both of us an overdose of tablets at the same time disguised in a drink, so that I could end her suffering and then end my life so that neither of us would live in my imagined nightmare any more. What a terrible thing to consider; what a terrible thing to write. I feel ashamed to admit that I have felt like that, but I have. When I think about those times now, I think that my reaction was all part of the shock, and the strong feeling that a mother has about protecting her children. I think that although I knew about the illness, and knew what to expect, the reality has sometimes been very difficult indeed. No mother imagines that they will watch their child suffer. You naturally want to protect them and make things better. When your child has a genetic illness you know that you are helpless. You know that your child will definitely suffer, and you won't be able to stop it.

We have lived with the illness for nearly seven years now. I have met other sufferers who are older and they are still living productive lives. I appreciate that no one can predict the severity or number of effects that Krystie will eventually experience. I also know that no matter what happens, that we will cope, and that Krystie will be happy. Time is a great healer, and it is a good teacher too. You have two choices: you can worry about everything and shut yourself away, or you can choose to make the best of everything and do as much as you can. That's what we have tried to do with Krystie.

She has always had access to information. I printed off information from the Internet and gave it to her to read. I always make sure that she gets to see the Ataxian newsletter. If she asks me a question I answer it. It would be true to say that she has known the broad picture from day one, but the detail has become apparent over the years. She has shown enormous maturity, is very brave and quite philosophical about everything. She explains that she doesn't dwell on yesterday, never worries about tomorrow and just enjoys every day. She has taught me a lot, and that 'degenerative' doesn't have to be scary.

Reality bites

6

Once I knew what we were dealing with, it was time to get on with it. In my mind I had sorted everything into a neat little order: Nicholas and Anthony were carriers like me; Harrison could be tested later; and Krystie had a strange illness.

The first thing that the medics did was to assess her body and record a baseline picture of how she was at the time of diagnosis. So a whole round of hospital appointments began. Amongst other things Krystie had to have a heart scan and her feet checked; it seemed that we were always at the hospital. We found out that both Krystie's feet and heart were already affected. The muscles of her feet were pulling against each other twisting her feet into awkward shapes. This meant that we visited a foot specialist called a podiatrist who took pictures of her feet and made a special sponge to sit in her shoes. She also had to be fitted for special shoes and trainers. As you can imagine, a young lady of nearly 10 was not at all happy about the prospect of wearing 'special' shoes. We searched the supplier's catalogues until Krystie found a model that she could feel comfortable in. We found out that her heart was enlarged on the left-hand side, causing an irregular heartbeat, but in the grand scheme of things we were told that her heart was in pretty good shape.

We were introduced to an occupational therapist and a physiotherapist; these were people who were assigned to our family, to provide support at home. The 'physio' was a lady called Jane Sellar who worked with Krystie to develop suitable exercises to help strengthen her muscles. She also provides advice on practical aids such as walking frames and wheelchairs. Jane still works with our family and has become a good friend. She has a good relationship with Krystie and understands her. She has been amazing in the support that she has provided using her medical knowledge to identify and anticipate changes. She has liaised with other specialists and provided everything that we have needed at just the right time.

When Krystie was in the last year of primary school, the year when you have reached the top of the tree and become the king of the school, so to speak, she faced a huge decision. She was becoming increasingly unsteady on her feet and would stumble into walls, radiators, people or just crash to the floor. It was very alarming. Both Jane and I agreed that she really needed to start using her wheelchair, but she would not listen. Finally the school expressed concern that she would seriously hurt herself or someone else when falling, so Krystie agreed to use a walking frame. Jane was keenly aware that this was very difficult for Krystie, and set about finding a frame that might appeal to a 10-year-old. She found a bright orange contraption called a Crocodile walker R82. Krystie had to stand in the middle of it and pull it behind her. You certainly couldn't hide it but it did the job of providing some stability around Krystie and enabled her to walk. Krystie was really worried about the reaction of her friends. She knew that she was going to stick out like a sore thumb, but she didn't have a choice. Her classmates found it all quite interesting and just accepted the change. Krystie coped by acting as if she were quite indifferent about it. Their reaction wasn't what she had expected, and she was glad about that. It must be really hard to face every day knowing that you are different, but she does it. Krystie also had a special helmet that she wore in the playground to protect her head when she fell. It looked like a riding hat; she chose a brown plaid design. It was padded with foam inside. She really did not like wearing that hat, but again for her own safety she accepted that it was the safest option. Her classmates didn't take too much notice; I think that she got teased a little, but it wasn't too bad. She also started to use chubby grip pens and pencils to help her grip, she appreciated that they helped her, but felt that they looked like nursery-type pens and pencils. She went through so much in such a short space of time. Ten years old is such a delicate time, when a child's confidence and self-esteem are being shaped; Krystie's self-image was being sorely tested.

Occupational therapists worked with us to look at the space of our home and advise us on any adaptations that we needed to make. They also provided practical aids that met the needs of specific problems. For example Krystie has an intention tremor on her hands, which basically means that when she uses her hands to cut her food or pick up a cup they shake. When she moves a fork or spoon towards her mouth her head shakes. So the occupational therapists advised us on special utensils. They provided Krystie with a rocker knife to make it easier for her to cut up food, and a beaker with a lid that has a hole for a straw. They also provided a plastic rim that fits to a plate forming a collar that allows Krystie to cut up her food without launching it into space (because of her jerky movements). Krystie was really not too happy about these things. She hates to be different; she feels that using these aids make her stand out, so whilst she might use them at home, she does not yet use them when we are out. I found it all unnerving. It's very hard to watch your children change so that they have to start using aids again. As mothers we all move our children through the infant stages of trainer cups and chunky cutlery and it is a milestone when they stop using them. I felt like Krystie was travelling in reverse and it didn't feel right. I could see the value and usefulness of the various items but I could easily understand how Krystie felt.

Between August 1999 (the time of diagnosis) and the following January was a time of meeting new people and finding out more about what was happening to Krystie's body. You almost didn't have time to really think about things, you just got on the treadmill. Alongside all of this I decided to look at alternative therapies.

Everything I read seemed to suggest that we could expect Krystie to be a full-time wheelchair user by the time she was 11. In addition, since she was already demonstrating multiple symptoms, and because of the early onset of the illness, it seemed that she had an aggressive form. I am a person who believes in the value of alternative therapies. I had experienced the benefit of them with my own hormone imbalance. I had struggled along using conventional medicine for many years not really making progress. It was only when I introduced alternative therapies and supplements that I really began to heal. So I took Krystie to visit a Dr Shamin Dyer in London in order to get her blood tested to check her mineral levels. I wanted to get her body in balance because it seemed reasonable to me that her own body at its optimum performance might be able to slow down the progression of the illness. So we got her blood tested and then gave her supplements to balance out her body.

I put her on a completely organic diet with no additives. I also took her to an interesting reflexologist in Rugby (Basil Cardew) on a regular basis. He said that he had had some success in treating a family with the same condition as Krystie. We would travel down to see him and he would massage her feet; she said that it hurt her quite a lot, but she thought that it was worth trying. During these months she did grow and she looked healthier. I also searched the Internet for any evidence of successful therapies. I couldn't find any. I looked at the information on disorders that seemed similar to hers, just to see if they were finding any useful therapies. I wrote to doctors who were having success in the treatment of illnesses like Parkinson's disease and CJD. In all cases I have found that doctors are very good at writing back to you. I haven't had a positive response (yet!); most explain that their treatment impacts a different nerve centre to that attacked by Friedreich's Ataxia, or they tell me that the route cause of the degeneration is different so they cannot help. They all wish us well. I looked into the medical centres in Mexico, but again could not find any evidence to suggest that they could really help Krystie. All of this activity is my way of coping. I fix things; I usually find a solution for everything. But not this time, I cannot do anything. I cannot make my daughter better, I just can't. As a mother this is a hard fact to accept.

I feel so sad about Krystie's illness. I had so many dreams for her. On the day that the diagnosis finally came through I faced the fact that those dreams would turn out very differently. As parents you always want the best for your children, you don't want to enforce anything on to them but you hope that they will face the world with energy. When you get news like we have had, everything freezes. It's like someone has taken a part of your hopes and dreams away. I felt that someone had played a trick on us. That we had thought for nine years of her life that she was fine, and then suddenly you realise the truth. It's a double blow. I look at her sometimes, and wonder how she copes. Most teenagers just enjoy each day and map out their lives; but from the age of 9 Krystie has had to know that her life would be (a) altered and (b) likely shortened. I admire her strength so much, because she just faces each day with resolution and spirit.

As a mother, I especially looked forward to the mother–daughter activities that I enjoyed as a teenager. Between the ages of 12 and 15 I used to go shopping in town with mom most Saturdays. We would walk arm in arm through the shops. I loved trying on clothes and shoes. Such a simple thing, but I cannot do that and never will with Krystie. Yes I know that I can still shop with her (and I do) but she is in her chair, and we cannot link arms. I cannot watch her twirl around in a shop changing room proudly modelling the latest fashion.

I have tried to be strong for Krystie. I have wanted her to be positive and not feel that her being around makes people sad. I have also tried to be strong for the boys. They have had their moments over the years. They have both cried to me in private, and shared their frustration and sadness. They have both questioned why ours should be the family with the illness. When Anthony decided to go travelling after his A levels he sat down with me one afternoon and said how he had thought about Krystie and wondered whether she would be able to do the same sort of things that he and Nicholas had been able to do. Who knows? None of us. Nonetheless we each need to live our lives and Krystie will live hers in the way she wants to I'm sure. As a mother it's difficult to watch your children suffering, you want their lives to be as carefree as possible. I also feel for my parents. They have lost their own son, and now they are watching their oldest granddaughter battle an illness. On top of this I know that they worry about me. I wonder sometimes why some families seem to have so much. So although I try not to cry at home, I have to let my grief out somewhere. I travel quite a lot with my job. When I am alone in my car, I get time to think. If I start to think about Krystie I can get upset. In the privacy of my car I cry, where there is no one to hear me and no one to see. Once I start crying I can cry for a very long time, so I'm glad that my journeys are often quite long. There are days when I think that I will never stop crying, ever. But you have to.

There have been a few public sessions of crying, which I absolutely hate, but can't stop, they just happen without warning. One occasion is very clear in my mind. It was very early September after her diagnosis; just a few days before the children went back to school. I took Krystie up to Beatties department store to buy some shoes. We walked in, took a number and sat down to take our turn. As we waited I was watching the other mothers and children. There were a couple of girls walking up and down steadily, sturdily and proudly. The assistant came and measured Krystie's feet, she returned with the shoes in her size range and tried the first pair on. Krystie started her ungainly walk across the store; the assistant shouted after her, 'Try and walk straight.' As she said it, I looked at her and said, 'That is her walk, she has a genetic illness that means she doesn't walk too well,' and then I just broke down and cried. The bewildered young girl didn't know what to do, she was apologising, and in between my sobs I was telling her not to worry. Other mothers glanced at me and then didn't know where to look. I was trying to stop crying because of Krystie being there. She came back and said, 'What's the matter mom?' I said, 'Nothing darling, don't worry sit down.' I was so annoyed with myself, and so embarrassed; but just for one day I wanted her to be like all the other children in the shop, I wanted her to walk strongly and proudly in her brand new shoes. She was never going to do that again. I felt so sad for her. I think that the emotion of the previous few months just cascaded out of me that day.

My eldest son Nicholas sums it up really when he says that you cope because you don't think about it, you just carry on, and that's so true. If you don't think too deeply about it you can cope. If you have times when you think about it, you just feel overpowered by emotion. It is too much, and you feel that you can't bear it. You can feel that you are going completely mad. You just want it to stop. Your breath feels short, and your chest feels tight. You want to wake up one morning and it's all been a dream. You want to give your child back their life. You want your children to have an equal chance; this drives you mad, it does. But you have to stop, you cannot afford to be engulfed by it; you just have to grit your teeth and get on with life.

People say, I don't know how you cope; you are so strong. But you are not, you don't feel it. What else can you do? Give up? Run away? You can't. You feel such a fraud, because you spend half your life silently screaming inside. You feel as if you are walking a tightrope, and so the only way to get through is to look straight ahead and take it steady. As the years have gone on, and the illness has made its insidious attack, I have felt that it sucks your energy. You have enough strength to get through each day, but you don't have much else left. I have come to realise that the emotional strain is very, very heavy. You get up each morning and you go to work, and school. You get through the day, and you welcome the rest at night, and then you get up the next day and do it again. I think that you sort of disconnect yourself, and function on a kind of autopilot, because it seems unreal, like you might be watching somebody else's life.

By the time Krystie was 10 she was really quite unsteady on her feet. She used a walking frame around school, and had to get used to standing out from the crowd. I remember that one day she came home from school upset that the assistants who managed the after-school club had told her that she could not use the climbing frame. When I went to talk to them about this, they were adamant that they would not take responsibility for her climbing the frame. I explained that I did not mind her climbing. She liked to sit on the first few rungs of the frame and because she wasn't standing could manage this really well. I said that I felt that she should be able to do as much as she wanted to, and that she never tried to do anything that felt difficult for her. They would not budge; they would not allow her to use it. I called her specialist, and the headmaster, both of whom felt that she should be allowed to use the equipment, but I could not persuade the assistants to change their minds. I don't think they realised the impact this had on Krystie. They did not try to see it from her point of view. This was our first taste of people's reactions to disability. Krystie was really upset by this and could not understand why they wanted to stop her using it. I remember her saying that she wouldn't be able to use it soon enough so why stop her now?

People would stare at her clumsy walking, or watch her using her walking frame. I explained that people were interested or curious, and probably didn't realise that they were staring, but Krystie still found it difficult.

Around this time Jane the physiotherapist told us about a drama group called the Fruit Cake Theatre Company. A student teacher ran it for a week during every school holiday. During the week the children learnt the songs, moves and dances and then at the end of the week they staged the performance. Krystie went along to one of these weeks and auditioned for a part in the *Lion King*. Krystie got the part of the wise old monkey Rafiki. She really enjoyed it, she had a great week. It was wonderful to watch her up on stage singing and dancing her heart out. She did really well. We captured it on film and I cried my eyes out. I was really proud of her, and it was so nice to see her happy and carefree. She returned to the group over the following months, and played La Fau in *Beauty and the Beast*, Mr Dawes in *Mary Poppins*, the Butler in *The Sound of Music* and finally Scarecrow in *The Wizard of Oz*. She wobbled all over the stage in her scarecrow outfit, which worked really well because she looked like she was playing a 'floppy scarecrow'. However, she decided that she wouldn't do any more plays after that one. She felt that it had really tired her out, and she had found it difficult to dance and keep her balance. But at least she had a taste of theatre if only for a few months. She was fantastic, and the experience was good for her confidence and self-esteem.

Krystie

Fruitcake Theatre was one of the most enjoyable things I've ever done, meeting new people, making new friends, dancing around, etc. Yeah, really fun. I fell over many times towards the end trying to do the dance moves. It was tiring but I loved it, and I wish I could go back and do it all again.

The first play I did was The Lion King. I was apprehensive beforehand. I could think of just over a million more interesting things I could be doing – but as soon as I got there, on the first day, I made friends. We had such a good time, laughing constantly. Jenny the organiser was really nice, and I'd often have a laugh with her and her friends. All I can say is that I miss those days.

I wanted her to build a bank of memories, so I encouraged her to do as much as she possibly could. We travelled to Mexico, and she swam with the dolphins, which she found exhilarating. I savoured every moment of watching her up on her feet enjoying her life; actually looking back I was building my memory bank too.

The Ataxia organisation contacted us to let us know that some doctors were running a drugs trial to find out whether high doses of vitamin C and co-enzyme Q10 could be beneficial to people who had ataxia. I talked to Krystie about helping out with the trials, because they really need children to take part in them. She could see the value in the research, and so decided to take part. She signed up for three years and agreed to be assessed every six months. It was yet another batch of hospital appointments to fit in, but we all felt that she should do it. She had to take several tablets every day. You don't know whether or not you have been given the true tablet or a placebo until the end of the trials. Some days she got fed up of taking the tablets (three years is a long time), and they made her feel sick. The doctors filmed her walking every six months, and recorded her results from manual dexterity tests (things like keyboard skills, and reacting to lights by pushing buttons in sequence). They also took pictures of her brain using MRI scans. Krystie didn't mind attending these clinic days; we attended hospitals in London, Cardiff and Liverpool. She was often reflective when we got home. This was because she would meet other people with the illness; and usually these people were older and more advanced in their symptoms. I would catch Krystie watching people and their jerky movements. These observations gave her a glimpse into her future and it shocked her. It stopped me in my tracks too. It is one thing to read about an illness and therefore be aware of it, but the reality is stark. Krystie's quietness on the way home, her guarded stares at people and her questions after each clinic visit told me that she was finding it hard to accept that she was eventually going to be similar to the people she saw. In her head I believe that she felt that her determination would drive her on forever. Therefore I think that these glimpses into the lives of others similarly afflicted were valuable in slowly preparing her for the future. They also prepared me.

The occupational therapists came again to look at our house to help us assess what, if any, adaptations we needed to make to accommodate Krystie. We had lived in the house for just over a year. It was a 1930s property, very nice, but was assessed as being fairly difficult to adapt. So we put the house up for sale and looked for a new place to live. We needed a house that could be easily adapted to provide a downstairs bedroom, and separate toilet and shower facilities. It was a nightmare trying to find something that could meet our needs. By now we had four children and that meant that we needed at least a four-bedroomed property with additional rooms downstairs that could be converted. We couldn't seem to find the right house within our price range.

Then I started to worry about Harrison and his closeness with Krystie. It was early in 2000 by now. Harrison was just over a year old. Amongst the jumble of my mind at that time was the recollection of the death of my own brother Andrew when I was 7 years old. I remembered very clearly how that felt. Krystie's life expectancy was (and is) uncertain. This was backed up by medical opinion and the experience of other Friedreich's Ataxia (FA) sufferers. Some people do live a relatively long life. However, the related medical problems that FA causes can reduce lifespan. In particular damage to the heart. We knew that Krystie's was already affected by the illness. She had cardiomyopathy of the left ventricle. The heart specialist explained that the function wasn't too bad really; in fact quite satisfactory, but FA can continue its attack at any time. I knew that quite a few sufferers had died of heart failure, including children.

I had a wide range of ages between my children. Nicholas was now 18, Anthony 16, Krystie 9 and Harrison was just 1. His closest sibling was Krystie. He loved all his brothers and sisters and they loved him too, but the boys were out and about a lot, socially and with part-time work, sports, etc., but Krystie was nearly always home. Harrison really identified with her. He focused on her. I couldn't imagine him getting so close to her and then if she died him being left alone. So I wanted to try for another baby. I was worried obviously because I knew that Krystie could become a full-time wheelchair user at any time. I understood that managing a wheelchair and a pushchair together would be a nightmare, but even so I just felt that I had to do it. I believed that we probably had just enough time to have a baby and get them through to toddler stage before Krystie would need to use a wheelchair full time. So after talking to Mitch about how I felt we decided to try for another baby. This meant looking for a house to accommodate seven people – talk about increasing the challenge!

Family ties 7

I was 38 by now, so not too old, but I did feel tired. We had all been through an enormous emotional trauma over the past twelve months, not to mention that Harrison had only just turned 1! Nevertheless, as always, I became pregnant easily. We were all delighted. I think that other people thought that we were mad, but you can't go round explaining your reasons can you?

I began to feel really concerned about whether or not the child I was carrying would be a boy or a girl. I didn't know which would be best, a boy for Harrison or another girl. I didn't want Krystie to feel like she was being replaced, and at the same time I knew in my heart that if anything happened to Krystie I would want another daughter, not to replace her, just because . . . I can't explain it . . . just because. Thinking about my mom, and her going back to having four children at home again, and because I would miss not having a girl if Krystie wasn't around, because you get used to what you have I suppose.

Krystie was still visiting Basil Cardew at this time for her reflexology sessions. Once he finished with Krystie, I used to have a little session to help my nerves. When I found out that I was pregnant, I called him to let him know that I wasn't feeling a 100 per cent and couldn't face the journey there and back each week (a 3-hour round trip) just at the moment. I told him my news by way of explanation. 'Really,' he said, 'you are pregnant?' 'Yes,' I said, 'I am.' 'Just one minute, let me open my computer because I want to check my notes from your last visit.' He opened his system and read his notes to me. 'Mrs Maddox – suspect she is pregnant, it's a girl.' I was completely shocked, because I must have only been about six to eight weeks at the time. 'You knew,' I said, 'How?' He said that he could tell by the blood rhythm and heartbeats. 'And you are sure it's a girl?' I asked him. 'Yes,' he said, 'it's a girl.' I told Mitch and no one else; I was really pleased. There was no point worrying now, the die was cast, as it were, but I did feel really happy.

About two months after this I had a scan at the hospital. I asked the scan operator if she could tell me what sex the baby was. She told us that she thought it was a boy. 'Are you sure?' I asked. 'Well it's got something a girl wouldn't have,' she replied. I was shocked. Mitch looked at me. I didn't know how to feel or what to believe. But later I decided to trust Basil. (You believe what you want to believe eh?) A few weeks later I took Krystie back to Basil and I told him what had happened at the hospital. 'Come on,' he said, 'let's have a look.' He sat and massaged away. 'Molvia, you are definitely carrying a little girl, I don't care what any scan machine has told you, it's a girl.' That was good enough for me. I knew I was carrying a girl. Then the worry started: How would Krystie feel? How would I feel? Had I done the right thing? Only time would tell.

I didn't tell anyone except Mitch about Basil. Mitch didn't know what to think. He was more inclined to trust the hospital scan; we agreed not to tell anyone else. I did however share the news with one other person, Jane Sellar, our physiotherapist.

I really like Jane – she's a mom like me, in fact her daughter is the same age as Krystie so I know she understands me. I know that she understands Krystie, and I know that she understands how I feel about things. We don't even have to talk; I just know that she knows. Jane popped in to see me to talk about Krystie and shoes. We sat at the kitchen table and I looked at her. 'Jane,' I said, 'I know what the baby is.' She looked at me expectantly. 'A girl,' I continued. As soon as I said it I just burst into tears, and tried to talk, 'I'm pleased and not pleased all at the same time, I don't know how to feel. Is it right to have another girl when your first girl is ill?' Jane shared my emotion; she understood exactly what I meant. 'Molvia, don't worry it will be fine.' And it was, well sort of.

Again I had a good pregnancy. I felt a bit tired, but I didn't have any of that awful sickness that I had experienced with my first three babies. However, at 36 weeks I developed severe haemorrhoids (piles), and I mean severe! I couldn't walk, sit down, stand up or lie down; I was in complete agony. I used the usual creams but nothing improved. I just got worse. My mom had to come and stay for a few days to help out because I simply couldn't move.

I visited the out-of-hours surgery at the weekend, and once the doctor examined me, he sent me straight to hospital. I was checked into a bed and told that a surgeon from the surgical ward would be asked to visit me (because I was on a maternity ward), but he never did. At every shift change the nurses would pop into my room to say, 'We've heard about your piles, we are not going to look at them though because we understand they're a bit grim, I'm sure you will be fine in a few days after a bit of rest.'

So basically instead of lying in my own bed I was now lying in a hospital bed. The only relief I got was from using a preparation called 'Instilagel' that anaesthetised the area. Only one midwife checked them during my stay; she was sympathetic but could only apply cream, she couldn't do anything else. After three days I was discharged. The midwife explained that they wouldn't do anything until after the baby was born, I only had around three weeks to delivery, and once the baby arrived they could do something (a small operation) but not before. Looking back I think that they thought that lots of pregnant women suffered with piles so I was just making a fuss. And of course it's true, I had had piles with all of my pregnancies, but nothing like these; I was distraught. I returned home, and my mom moved in to look after everyone.

I have never felt such an intense pain in my whole life. After a couple of days literally lying in bed crying I could take no more. I telephoned my obstetrician's secretary and begged her to book me into clinic to see him. I explained why. I was clearly upset, so she arranged for me to visit him at his next clinic in two days' time. Somehow, I drove myself to the hospital and walking like a complete idiot I got to the clinic. The specialist remembered me from Harrison's birth. 'Oh hello Mrs Maddox; I understand that you have problems with piles. Come on then, let's have a look at you.' I lay on the couch and he examined me. 'Good God, woman,' he said, 'you have to see a surgeon today.' He telephoned across to the surgical ward and spoke to a surgeon telling him that he was sending me over to see him immediately. I cried with relief that someone was going to do something. I knew that the pain that I was experiencing wasn't right. It transpired that my piles were strangulated and infected; if I had taken the advice of the maternity ward and done nothing until the baby's birth (another three weeks away) then we might not have actually made it.

The surgeon explained that I was in serious danger of the infection developing into something much more serious, and against his usual practice he was going to have to remove the piles as soon as possible even though I was so heavily pregnant. I begged him to let me go home to ensure that the children and everyone were sorted out. I then returned to the hospital the next day.

Once I was admitted they monitored me for a couple of days and scheduled the surgery. By now I was 36/37 weeks pregnant. I was terrified of what would happen to my precious baby girl. I requested that they deliver McKenna by Caesarean and then remove the piles, because the most important thing to me was that she was delivered safely. However, the medics would not agree to this. My obstetrician said that I should remember what happened to Harrison, and that a baby's lungs at 36 weeks were just not predictable. In his opinion the baby was better off staying in my womb until it reached full term, 40 weeks. He explained that the surgeon would use a spinal block to anaesthetise me to allow him to remove the piles and that I would then have a couple of weeks to heal before delivering McKenna at full term. I could not imagine how they expected me to deliver a baby vaginally once the piles had been surgically removed. It just didn't make sense, but I bowed to their combined experience and agreed to their plan. The other slight worry I had was in connection with the spinal block. I remembered the reaction to it when I had delivered Harrison, but the surgeon assured me that I would be fine. On the morning of the surgery, the anaesthetist came to see me. She was visibly shocked to find out that I was heavily pregnant. She explained that no one had told her that I was pregnant, and bluntly said that she would not be held accountable for the well-being of my baby. I was feeling more distressed by the minute, and wanted to know what she meant. She said that in her opinion I was putting the baby at risk. Well, I just started to cry, I was frightened to death. In between sobs, I told her that I had begged them to deliver my baby first. She agreed that this was the safest option. By now I was inconsolable, and said that I would not have the surgery. The nurses fetched the surgeon. He came to see me and was clearly annoyed with me. He asked me why I was wasting his time by refusing the operation. His irritation surprised me, but crystallised everything in my mind. I very calmly touched his arm, held his jacket sleeve, and said, 'My daughter at home, my only daughter is 10. She was diagnosed with an incurable genetic condition just over a year ago. I do not know how long I am going to have her.' Touching my belly I continued, 'This child in here is another daughter, I will not risk losing her too; and your anaesthetist has just stood next to me and told me that I am putting her at risk. I will not do it. My priority is this child. Deliver her, and then sort out my piles.' The tears were glistening in my eyes, and my voice was full of emotion but I spoke calmly. He looked at me and instantly understood; he visibly softened. 'Alright Mrs Maddox, I am going to fetch your obstetrician to come and talk to you. We will see what he has to say, but your baby will be fine, I assure you of that.' My obstetrician came and listened to me, but would not budge. He did not agree with the anaesthetist and felt that the baby would be fine. He did, however, promise me that he would stand by my side during the procedure and if the baby seemed to get into distress that he would deliver her immediately. So I agreed to go ahead and went down to theatre. As they wheeled me down, I felt very scared about the spinal block, but no one seemed to think that it was going to be a problem. I didn't feel that they were being logical. I would have felt much happier delivering McKenna and then taking away the piles. I just did not believe that I would be able to push a baby out after having had surgery on my back passage!! No one listened. With some trepidation I had the spinal block and lay down. After a few minutes that strange familiar feeling started in my head. I looked up at the anaesthetist and said, 'My head's going funny again, it's just like Harrison.' 'Oh, Mrs Maddox you are fine, don't worry, you're just nervous,' she said looking down at me. 'No,' I started, 'No, this is jus. . . .' I was gone. The next thing I remember was someone slapping my leg, while someone else was talking loudly and urgently into my ear, 'Molvia, Molvia, Wake up!' As I started to regain some focus, I was aware that someone else was shouting, 'Get him back. Fetch him now!' At the same time someone was propping me up and tapping me. I found out later that the obstetrician had indeed watched them administer the spinal block, but because I initially seemed all right he had slipped out of the room telling them that I would be fine. However, I had suffered that strange reaction to the spinal block again and lost consciousness. The anaesthetist was looking at me very concerned; I smiled weakly at her, and said, 'I told you that I felt odd again.' 'I know love,' she said, 'I know.' The surgeon said 'Keep her propped up and let's get this done as quickly as possible.' The obstetrician stood by me, and they cauterised the piles. I was taken back to the ward. I felt stressed and upset but glad to be alive, and most of all glad to have a live baby inside me. I was discharged just two days later. It was a Saturday afternoon. I got home at lunchtime. At approximately two o'clock the telephone rang. It was the hospital. Mrs Maddox, could you come into hospital on Wednesday in preparation for a Caesarean section on Thursday. I couldn't believe it, 'What?' I exclaimed, 'But he told me that I would have a normal delivery. I begged him, I begged him.' I couldn't believe it. 'Yes Mrs Maddox, but after watching the surgery the other day, he does not want you to undergo a vaginal delivery.' I couldn't believe it. I had expressed that concern myself a number of times (and I'm not a doctor!), but no one listened. Now I had another worry – the spinal block. Not a third one, surely not. I thought that I would die on the operating table. I kept thinking about people who have reactions to things, and how in some cases the reaction gets stronger each time it occurs. This would be my third spinal block; I could remember the strange feeling it gave me in my head and felt sick with worry. I had four children at home, but my main concerns were Harrison, Krystie and this unborn baby. If anything happened to me what would happen to them? What about my new little girl, what if I never ever saw her? With pregnancy hormones rife in my system, my fears felt very real. I was a very scared woman indeed.

I went into hospital, and when the anaesthetist came to talk to me on the evening before the operation she explained that the spinal block seemed to do its job very very well on me. That is, instead of numbing my system to just above my tummy button, it travelled very high, and that is why it had affected my heart. However, now they understood what was happening they intended to monitor me very closely. They also intended to perform the Caesarean with me in a semi-upright position so that the spinal block would not travel up my system quite so quickly. She also said that I was first on the next day's operating list and that the most senior person in every discipline would be supporting the operation. 'You have the top team, Mrs Maddox, you will be fine,' she said. I felt a little more confident, but still worried.

They once again administered the spinal block. After a few minutes my head started to feel a bit strange. The anaesthetist was watching me like a hawk; she pulled me completely upright and then injected my arm. 'Come on,' she said, 'Lets get this baby out as quickly as possible.' I didn't lose consciousness, but I felt odd. I had the Caesarean with me sitting propped up in a near upright position, but our daughter was delivered safely. My second daughter McKenna Joni-Mae Maddox arrived. I cried and cried.

She was healthy and beautiful; we took her home. Krystie loved her; she was so pleased to have a sister. She didn't seem in any way shape or form jealous of her, so it had worked out after all.

We returned home on about 12 November. My family felt complete. My older children loved the 'little ones', and the little ones loved their big brothers and sisters. I had three sons and two daughters, what a blessing. I think that we all felt tied together, threaded together by the babies.

Krystie

Harry and Kenna: the rugrats. Well of course I love them, though I find them extremely annoying, most of the time. When they first arrived, I'll admit it, I was jealous of them. I was used to being the baby of the family, and hated the fact that everything changed suddenly.

It doesn't bother me now though, although they still bug the hell outta me when they come in my room and mess with my stuff. They're good kids though and I love them unconditionally whether they're annoying me or not; and I always will. I love all my family to be honest and can't imagine life without any one of them. I had an operation not long ago and when I came out of hospital the kids were on holiday, and I didn't feel like I was home until they got back. I'd miss them if they weren't there. What can I say, they're my brother and sister.

We had managed to both sell and find a new house during the pregnancy. The move date was set for early December just a few weeks away. I was in a very emotional state. The last few weeks of my pregnancy had been very stressful and now here I was fresh out of a Caesarean section with two babies, a poorly daughter and a house move to manage. Mitchell was working really hard. He hated me being pregnant, really didn't like it at all. The worry over my last few weeks had really got to him and we were both just far too tired to cope with moving house. He could go off to work each day, but I was at home gingerly trying to pack with a great big healing scar across my tummy. It was a very difficult time. The solicitors finally got their act together to enable us to move house on 20 December.

We were really pleased with the new house. It had an extra sitting room downstairs which was next door to a large downstairs toilet. We intended to use this room as a ground floor bedroom for Krystie, and then convert the toilet into a wet room. The house also had an indoor swimming pool built in a separate wing off the kitchen. This was the room that clinched the deal for us. One of the doctors had told Krystie that she needed to keep mobile as long as possible. Quite simply he said, 'Krystie use it or lose it!' We felt that if she could swim most days that it would help her mobility and maintain her ability to walk for a bit longer. The thing was that buying the house stretched us financially to the limit, at a time when I was planning to take the next year off work in an extended maternity break. Mitchell really felt under pressure.

Mitchell had gone through a lot of change really. He was a bachelor when I met him with no responsibilities; and although we hadn't rushed into anything, once we had got married everything happened at break-neck speed. In the three years following the wedding, we had worked and lived in America, returned to the UK, started a consultancy business, bought a house, sold it and bought a second one, and also added two children to our family. Mitchell had to learn how to be a dad overnight almost. On top of this, he had to come to terms with the news about Krystie. Mitch is a typical man; he doesn't like to show his emotions, and likes to fix things. Throughout Krystie's illness he had agreed to pay for all of the alternative treatments that we pursued; he spent time like me searching the Internet for cures and treatments. He had accompanied us to some hospital appointments and been generally supportive. But in his head, he was going to find a cure, and if we remained positive then Krystie would be fine. The problem was that we couldn't fix this, no one could. As her mother although I find it hard to watch her deteriorate and want to help her maintain her independence I know when the time has come to accept a change. It is true to say that initially it is embarrassing taking a wheelchair out, you do feel like everyone is looking at you. You do also feel that everyone thinks your child automatically has mental problems. You feel so protective of their image. Every parent I'm sure will understand what I mean when I say that you feel a sense of pride to watch your children grow up strong. Just watching them walk into a room and knowing that other people look at them and think that they are lovely makes you feel proud. However, when people see a wheelchair they don't quite know what to do, they look away quickly, or stare, or look sympathetic. You don't want that reaction, you just don't. Then there are the other people who speak over the child to you in those cooing tones. It's not pleasant. Mitchell is basically a shy person; he hates being the centre of attention. So being out and about with Krystie with her visible problems has been a massive adjustment for him. There have been times when the friction between us has been difficult. He has explained to me that when we got married he accepted the fact that we didn't have the time that most couples get when you are just the two of you on your own, but he always expected that we would enjoy time together later on in life. The nature of Krystie's illness has meant that in his mind he doesn't see us having that time. I don't think that you can worry about the future; we will have to deal with that once it arrives. But his fears have meant that sometimes he has seemed irritated by the changes. Also, the extra planning that is necessary before you can do anything with a wheelchair. That irritation, not always recognised by anyone else, has been like a thorn in my side, because he is the one person that I would want to feel supported by. In his own way, he has been really excellent, and I know that even men who are the children's natural parents can find the challenges of chronic illness and disability difficult. I just think that the pressure has tested our relationship, and at times cost us the closeness that we once shared.

When Harrison and McKenna were younger it was very difficult juggling everything. For example, during 2001 Krystie had hospital appointments nearly every three weeks. Can you imagine taking a toddler, a baby and a clumsy 10-year-old all over the country? We did have times when we had appointments every single week. I also had Nicholas studying for A levels and Anthony studying for GCSEs. I was trying to cater for all my children's needs. In those early days (after diagnosis) I wasn't really emotionally strong about everything myself. I was still coming to terms with the reality of the illness. I felt like I was on a state of high alert, constantly checking that Krystie was coping with everything. It was difficult trying to protect her from herself at times.

Krystie is fiercely independent. She was really fed up with all the hospital appointments. She didn't want 'funny' shoes and trainers. She hated using her crocodile walker. She got sick of going to alternative practitioners, and didn't want to take advantage of the therapies that were on offer by the health authority either. She just wanted to be a 10-year-old. I used to try and put myself in her shoes and understand how she felt. She knew that her family was sad about the illness. Her grandparents, uncles, aunts, cousins, brothers and sisters. Just about everyone close to you is affected. As you can imagine, for a time everyone wanted to know about the illness. You would try not to talk when she was within earshot, but children are not stupid. She hated 'that' kind of attention. She was determined to prove that she was still OK. So she simply refused to use her crocodile walker except when she was at school. She wouldn't use her wheelchair if we went shopping. She preferred to hold onto my arm and walk close to me. I would take her weight and practically hold her up. It started to impact what I could do with her. At about this time an article in one of the Sunday magazines caught my eye. It was about a doctor called Mosaraf Ali. He was an alternative practitioner who used a lot of massage. I made contact with him, and took Krystie along to see him. He was based in New Cavendish Street, London, so again it was a bit of a trek, but I felt that his treatment might be beneficial.

He taught me how to massage her legs and other parts of her body, in particular he paid close attention to the area at the top of her spine and the base of the skull. He explained that this area was called the cerebellum and was linked to the pituitary gland and hypothalamus of the brain. When we first started to see him Krystie was still very small, she was by now 10 but was still wearing age 6/7 clothing. She carried no weight and was so petite. He felt that his massage would help her balance, which was getting worse, and he also commented on her growth (or lack of it). He was a lovely man, very calm. I trusted him, and so we started to visit him once a month.

So, it was quite a busy time and then just when you think that things can't get any worse it was time to think about Krystie's transfer to secondary school.

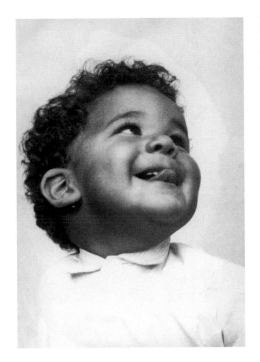

Molvia's brother, Andrew Williams, at 2½. He died of complications after measles, aged 5

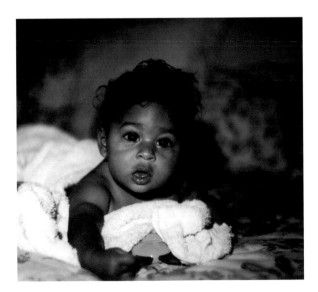

Krystie at 3 months

In 1991 with her faithful
friend 'Dancer'

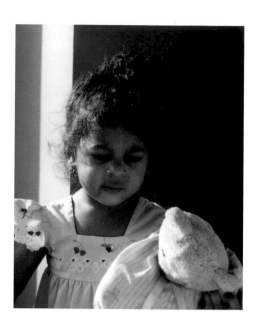

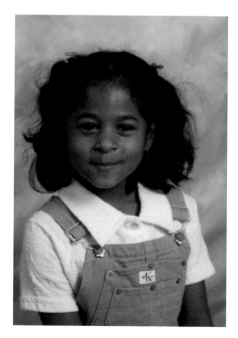

Krystie's American school
photo

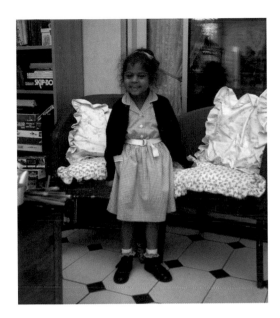

Aged 6. She is starting
to develop her own
way of standing

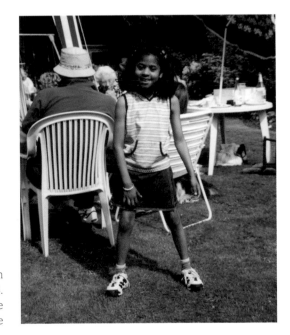

At a garden party in
the spring of 1998.
Again, notice
her stance

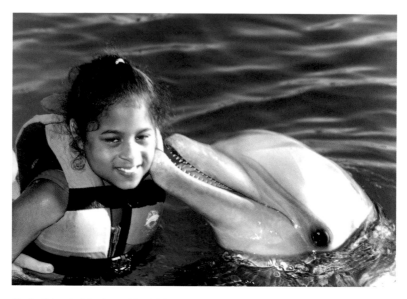

On holiday in Mexico with dolphins in December 1999

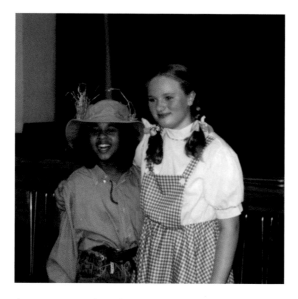

As a scarecrow in a play, summer 2002

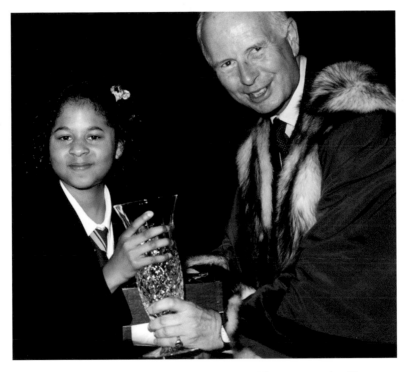

Aged 12, receiving the Emma Shaw personality of the year award at Thomas Telford School (courtesy of D.J. Houlston photography)

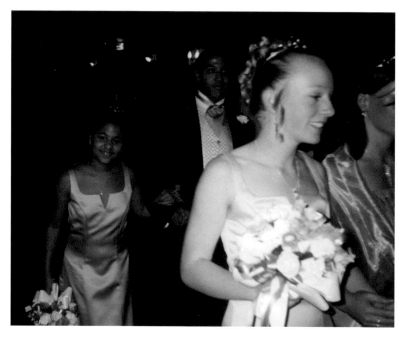

As a bridesmaid walking on her brother Anthony's arm, September 2003

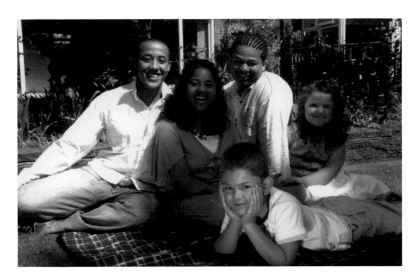

Krystie with her brothers and sisters, July 2005

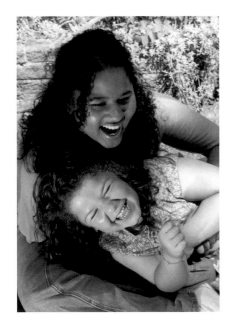

Krystie and McKenna, July 2005

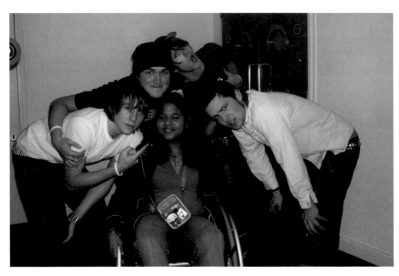

Meeting Mcfly in May 2005

Getting an education 8

Like all children of 10, it was time to consider which secondary school to apply for. My eldest son Nicholas attended a school called Thomas Telford. It is a city technical college, one of the top performing schools in the country. Anthony had won a scholarship to a local independent school, so educationally they were both well catered for. I didn't envisage providing anything less for Krystie.

I didn't think that she would be able to manage at the independent school. It is based in an old historic and very beautiful building, but is not suitable for wheelchairs. So the only local school that I felt would give her the type of education that I wanted for my children was Thomas Telford.

One of the many things that had happened during the previous year (2000) was that Krystie was 'educationally statemented'. I wasn't happy about the decision to take Krystie through the process at first, because I felt that there was nothing wrong with her learning abilities. I hadn't appreciated that statements are put in place to protect the child no matter what kind of challenges they may face. A statement is a document drawn up by the school, an educational psychologist and any other related medical personnel that can have a valuable input. So in Krystie's case, because her challenges are physical, Jane Sellar had an input as the physiotherapist, and an occupational therapist was also involved. An educational statement can be a lengthy document. It records the child's particular challenge, and describes the nature of any medical condition. It takes into consideration the likely progression of the illness or condition and makes recommendations for how the child can best be supported to enable them to achieve the best that they possibly can. It is a living document so is reviewed annually. In Krystie's case, the statement talked about Friedreich's Ataxia, and what the condition means. It explained why the condition means that Krystie has special educational needs. The objectives of the statement were recorded as follows:

- Maintain her independence for as long as possible
- Maintain her high academic standards and achieve her educational potential
- Participate meaningfully and purposefully in all curricular activities to the limits of her physical capabilities
- Access the National Curriculum at levels that are appropriate for her age and aptitudes.

I felt that these objectives were beneficial to Krystie. The document also discusses practical considerations, for example toilet facilities, wheelchair access, transport and any physical support that might be required. So it is what it says it is, a comprehensive statement of your child's particular needs. It provides a point of reference for everyone involved in support- ing your child.

Once you have a statement, you must declare it when applying for a school place. This was the problem.

Every family who has a child in year 6 receives a booklet that lists the schools that you can choose from when your child makes the transition from primary to secondary education. When our booklet arrived it listed the fourteen state schools within our catchment area. Included in this number were details of Thomas Telford with a note to explain that Thomas Telford is classified as a city technical college. This means that it operates independently of the local education authority (LEA), more like an independent school but is non-fee paying. It is sponsored jointly by the Tarmac group and the Mercers' Company and opened in 1991. It is an excellent school, which achieves high results across all ability bands winning national acclaim and is regarded as being an example of successful education methods. Its mission statement is: to raise education standards through effective practice and share it. The headmaster, Mr Satchwell, has been knighted for his services to educa- tion. It is a modern school, which is well equipped to meet the needs of wheelchair users, and provide support for individual needs.

Nicholas was attending this school. He is dyslexic, but achieved good results despite his challenges. I wanted Krystie to go there too.

It is a very difficult school to get into. It is massively oversubscribed, and is set up to take approximately 60 per cent of its intake from Telford where it is based, and the other 40 per cent from Wolverhampton where we live. However, this percentage breaks down further because all children who apply to the school have to sit entrance tests. The test scores are analysed by computer to select children across all ability bands. It takes the highest percentage of pupils from the average band, but also takes high-flyers and children who are lower achievers. The school does not guarantee to take siblings, so just because Krystie had a brother at the school did not guarantee her a place. We knew this was true, because Anthony had applied for a place at the school but was unsuccessful. Fortunately, he won his scholarship to Tettenhall College and was very happy there.

We completed the relevant forms and dutifully noted that Krystie had an educational statement. I enclosed a copy for their inspection. Encouragingly, Krystie was invited to take the entrance test, so we waited for the day to arrive. I wasn't too worried about the tests, but then it wasn't me sitting them (as Krystie reminded me)! Krystie's statement classified her as an above average achiever, so I expected that she would probably do well. The only drawback was that if this was the case, her percentage chance of gaining a place at the school was even smaller! She sat the tests and then had to wait several weeks to find out if she had been successful or not. Finally the letter arrived to say that one of the senior teachers wanted to talk to me. I nervously contacted the school, who explained that they very much wanted to offer Krystie a place, however they had noticed that Krystie was 'statemented' for special needs and therefore they were a little concerned as to whether or not Wolverhampton would fund the statement for her to attend Thomas Telford. It seemed that although Thomas Telford was listed in the Wolverhampton schools brochure, technically it was viewed as more like an independent school. Furthermore it was actually sited out of town, so if a child had special needs it presented a problem because the Wolverhampton LEA could refuse to fund the statement, preferring you to attend a school within the Wolverhampton borough. This meant that before Thomas Telford could give us a firm offer of a place we had to ensure that Wolverhampton LEA would indeed fund the statement.

Krystie had taken the tests in October and now it was either late November or early December, I can't quite remember. We both felt like we had been waiting forever to find out if she had won her much longed for place. The news that we received was bittersweet, and uncertain. Krystie was both pleased and nervous at the same time. She didn't know whether to laugh or cry. I was in the middle of a house move, with two young children under 2, and didn't know if I had the strength to battle. I also felt very angry. Just because Krystie had this illness it was possible that she was going to miss out on attending one of the best schools in the country; after everything that she had been through it seemed so unfair.

I contacted the local education authority to discuss the situation. They told me bluntly that it was unlikely that they would agree to Krystie attending Thomas Telford. They suggested that they had a perfectly adequate school within the city that had a unit for wheelchair users (Krystie's statement noted that the healthcare professionals felt that Krystie's use of a wheelchair was imminent) and that Krystie could attend there instead! They could not offer me a place at any other Wolverhampton school because of the anticipated use of a wheelchair. I was really upset; the school that they recommended had failed its Ofsted report and had been placed on special measures. Talk about complete opposites; the gulf between the two schools was enormous. I was devastated. To make matters worse, the school in question was on the opposite side of town to our home, and if Krystie had not been expected to soon become a wheelchair user was not a school that anyone attended from our area.

I felt like they were choosing her school on the basis of her disability, and that Krystie Maddox-Lue had disappeared to be replaced by a wheelchair. Already they were not seeing a person, just a piece of equipment. I was absolutely disgusted. I wrote to the LEA voicing my concerns, and explaining in no uncertain terms that I would not accept a place at the school of their choice. I was hormonal, and very upset, but I was determined that I would not give in. They basically said that I had two choices: (1) accept the school that they were offering and have it named in the statement; (2) name no school in the statement and enter into an informal agreement with Thomas Telford. This meant that we would in effect send her to Thomas Telford with no responsibility falling upon Wolverhampton LEA except for them to maintain the statement (not fund it). Thomas Telford had already stated that they would not do this.

The law said that I should be able to exercise parental preference. However, Wolverhampton were effectively giving me no choice. They were insisting that Krystie attend the school that they suggested. I told Krystie not to worry and explained to her that I was going to fight the education department on this matter. As far as I was concerned she was now in the unfortunate situation that out of a class of 34 children, she was the only child that did not know which secondary school she was going to attend in September. She couldn't join her friends in the excited chatter about their new schools, so not only was she separated from them in the playground by her walking frame, but she couldn't even join in the school conversations on this the current hot topic. She was really upset, and understandably worried. Not one child from her school was going to transfer to the school on offer to her, whilst two children in her class were going up to Thomas Telford.

I contacted the Department for Employment and Education in Westminster and spoke to them about our position. They explained that a new bill was due to be introduced in 2001 called the Special Educational Needs and Disability Bill. This bill was designed to protect families experiencing our sort of difficulties. They told me that most authorities were trying to work in the spirit of that bill in advance of its becoming law. They also advised me to speak to the Tribunal offices for their view and if necessary I could escalate my grievance to them. I contacted the Tribunal offices for a preliminary discussion. They said that in their opinion it was unreasonable for Wolverhampton LEA to state that they would only maintain the statement. They said that if an education authority maintains a statement then they also have a responsibility to follow up and ensure that the needs in the statement can be met. This obviously meant that they should be prepared to make some funding provision. More importantly they advised me that if I did decide to take the case to appeal that it would take approximately four months to reach a decision. In our case this meant that the case would not be concluded until October. This placed us in the intolerable position whereby Krystie was at risk of not being able to take up her secondary school place (at any school) in September. This put her at risk of missing the vital first few weeks when bonds are formed and firm friendships made. I did not want her to be placed in that position.

It was May 2001 now and I sat down and wrote a detailed letter explaining our situation and arguing for Krystie to be allowed to take up her place at Thomas Telford. I really did not want to go through the lengthy appeal process; it was imperative that she start the new school year on the first school day in September. I thought long and hard before crafting that letter. I referred to the new Bill that I had been told about and also hinted at the fact that it was her basic *human* right to have access to a good standard of education. I wanted anyone who read that letter to know in no uncertain terms without my actually threatening it that I would take this case to the European Court of Human Rights if necessary. I copied the letter to the Wolverhampton LEA, Thomas Telford, Krystie's then current head teacher, the medics who looked after her, the education office at Westminster and all of our local councillors. Then I sat back and waited.

One July afternoon, during the last but one week of term, I took a telephone call from the LEA. They called me to say that they had decided to name Thomas Telford in the statement. It was an eleventh-hour reprieve. Krystie had gone through her last primary school year without knowing where she was going to be next, which was a shame. But I felt jubilant to be able to tell her that we had won, and that she could take up her place at Thomas Telford. She was ecstatic; she deserved it. It was one of the happiest days of my life. Our determination had paid off. We could enjoy the summer

Krystie

Thomas Telford School. I remember the battle that mom had trying to make it possible for me to go there. Actually thinking about this makes me realise just how much mom has done for me, and continues to do. At the time I didn't realise just how much she was doing just to keep me happy. Thanks mom. But yes, there were many letters and phone calls, I know that much. I never actually read a letter, or listened properly to a call, but I heard snippets, and I'd hear mom come back from the office and rant about something or other. I really wanted to go to TTS mostly because my brother had gone there and enjoyed himself, and because it was and is the best comprehensive school in the country, not that I fully understood the significance of that back then. I can't remember the day that I found out I'd got in, but I do know that I was ecstatic. Finally I'd been accepted, how lucky was I. One battle over, bring on the next!

Krystie started her new school on the first day of term like everyone else. She was a little apprehensive about everything. She had been protected at her primary school, and had been with children who had known her since nursery school. This meant that they knew her before the illness. Krystie had managed to get by with a walking frame at primary school, but now she was worried that strangers would take one look at the bright orange frame and write her off. She flatly refused to use it. I could not persuade her; Jane could not persuade her. She stubbornly refused point blank to use it at Thomas Telford. She said that if she concentrated really hard that she could walk by herself. She had been having the massage by Dr Ali and was also swimming most days. Maybe all of this had strengthened her muscles or maybe it was pure bloody-mindedness! I don't know, but whatever it was she seemed able to walk a little stronger. She would not wear her protective hat or have any help. Jane told me that this was quite remarkable; she explained that Krystie uses much more energy just trying to do the simplest task. The fact that she was now walking around a large secondary school and was managing a longer school day was incredible.

Despite Krystie's bravado, I think that she found some things a little bit difficult. Secondary schools are large, and there are lots more people, people who are in a hurry and far too busy to make allowances for anyone who moves at a slower pace. But the only concession that Krystie made was that she decided to go into the library at break times rather than face the playground. She used to help the librarian. The school is very well organised, and the staff kept a watchful eye over her. Thomas Telford employs classroom assistants who are available to help children who have challenges. Krystie was not the only person who had either physical or learning difficulties and so the assistants formed a pool of support, and went to help various children at set times. They helped Krystie at lunchtimes. She has a tremor in her hands, which becomes apparent whenever she puts the muscles under pressure to do things. So, for instance, holding a pencil is a fairly light task, so although her hands might shake a little they are not too bad. If she holds a cup or a plate, the increased weight means that the tremor is more pronounced. When she tried to carry her lunch tray – well, look out anyone in the vicinity! With her arms both being outstretched at the same time, bearing weight whilst trying to walk, it was a disaster waiting to happen. Everyone quickly realised that the safest option was to ask an assistant to accompany her to the lunch queue and carry her tray for her. Krystie, her independence threatened again, was not amused. She said that she felt like she was being made to look like a baby. This self-image that she was starting to create in her head was not helped because she was still very small.

I remember that her school trousers were age 7. Krystie was nearly 11, and her trousers were that small! Krystie was feisty and quite prepared to stick up for herself, but she told me that she felt like people thought she was bit strange. She knew that her movements were jerky sometimes, and her walk was not quite right. Now having an adult carry her lunch tray was all just a little too public. Even though she protested, she knew that it was for the best. Like a lot of other things she really didn't have a choice, she just had to put up with it. In spite of everything she seemed happy, and settled in well at her new school.

When she arrived home from school each day I noticed that she was very tired, and that immediately she used her walker for support. This meant that she must have been really pushing herself to cope with the school day. Jane was always looking for ways to help Krystie and came to see us about a therapy that was being successfully used in Australia called 'Second Skin'. It was a skintight suit that was boned. Each person who uses one is filmed by a special computer and a suit is developed that is built to fit the muscular structure of that particular person. The science of it is that by gripping the muscles tight, the messages can be directed along the nerve pathways more smoothly, and therefore you can prolong the ability to walk for longer. We attended yet another clinic, and met the doctors who fitted Krystie for her own second skin. She chose a front panel that depicted blue dolphins. She was not thrilled at the prospect of wearing the suit under her uniform, especially in the summer, but she agreed to give it a go. The suit was duly made, and she went along for a fitting. They look a little bit like wetsuits. It was so tight fitting that it was a real effort to get Krystie into it! She hated the fact that she had to be dressed in it and couldn't put it on independently, but she did wear it, and it did help her walk more steadily.

It seemed like we had just managed to help Krystie keep on her feet when a flu virus struck her down. Krystie's immune system is not very strong. If she catches a cold, it can really knock her for six. She took to her bed, and was off her feet for just over a week. When she got better and tried to walk, she found that she just didn't have the same muscle strength. It was no good; she was going to have to use her walking frame at school again. It was around Easter time, so she had been at the school for a couple of terms. She was mortified, but even though Krystie is stubborn she is also very sensible. No one had to tell her that she had to use the walking frame; she recognised the fact herself. Once again her classmates thought that the frame was quite interesting, but they didn't really take too much notice, much to her relief. I was so proud of Krystie; my heart went out to her. I knew how much it had meant to her to be able to walk around her new school by herself, and yet after only a few months her dream had been shattered.

I was at home one day when the *This Morning* television programme asked people to phone in if they wanted to nominate someone for a treat. I thought about Krystie. We had been in the new house for about six months now. Krystie was sleeping in what had previously been a second ground-floor sitting room. It was very pink (which Krystie being a tomboy hated!), very long and narrow, and didn't really look like a young girl's bedroom. I thought that it would be fabulous if the programme could make over the room for her. I picked up the phone and after several attempts managed to get through on the nomination line. I recorded my message about Krystie and waited. Within half an hour someone had called me back to talk to me about my nomination. They listened to my story, and said that they would like to send a researcher out to meet us both. Emma came to see us a few days later. She had a chat with Krystie and as she left told me that she really liked Krystie, but would have to go back to the studios and have a chat with the producers before the final decision could be made. Why does everything involve waiting? But once again, the waiting paid off! Just a few days later I took a call from Emma to say that Krystie had been successful, and that Stephanie Dunning, the interior designer, would be coming to make over Krystie's bedroom. I could not wait for Krystie to return home from school so that I could share the news with her.

When I told her, she could not believe it. 'It's because of my Friedreich's, mum. They say every cloud has a silver lining, don't they?

If I didn't have Friedreich's they wouldn't be making my bedroom over, and I wouldn't get a chance to appear on the telly!' Her face was beaming; as she spoke she was brimming with childish happiness. I hadn't expected that kind of comment and was really choked. Krystie had her own particular take on life, and her own way of seeing things; you couldn't help but love her for it. The TV crew arrived and over the course of three mad days made over her bedroom. Stephanie the designer was a lovely lady. She seemed genuinely fond of Krystie, and explained to me that she used to be a physiotherapist so knew exactly what Krystie's condition meant for the future. She was only too pleased to be able to manage the makeover for us. With Krystie's condition in mind, she laid a laminate floor, and widened the doorway so that her bedroom would be more accessible for Krystie's wheelchair in the future. The finished design was absolutely beautiful. Krystie was almost speechless when she saw it. The resulting film was broken down into four parts and screened over four days during the Ideal Home week on TV. Thomas Telford also aired it on the internal TV loop. Krystie felt like a mini celebrity. I was pleased that I had been able to arrange the experience for her; her smiling face was worth it. When I watch the video of the programme now, it's hard to realise just how small and unsteady she looked at that time. The strangest thing is to watch her on her feet, I have to think really hard to think of Krystie walking; how soon you forget.

Krystie

Lights. Camera. Action. My television debut, that was possibly one of the most exciting times of my life. There's not really much I can tell you except how excited I was. I wasn't at all worried about going on tele, simply happy that I was going to be on a very popular breakfast programme. I remember going to school the day after they did filming. The second I walked into the lesson I was bombarded with questions. I felt so special. Not that I don't always, teehee. Thought I'd had my fifteen minutes of fame after that. How wrong was I?

Krystie continued to visit Dr Ali for her massage, and almost without us noticing Krystie started to grow. Quite unexpectedly, one school morning, her trousers were impossibly tight. We somehow managed to squeeze her into them, and during that day I went to buy her some new ones. Just three weeks later, the same thing happened again, and then just a few weeks after that it happened again. It was incredible. Krystie had never seemed to grow (not so you'd notice anyway!). Her clothes and shoes seemed to fit her for years, they really did. During that summer she had one of her appointments with Dr Anderson. As usual, the nurses recorded her weight and height. The nurse had to check the results three times before writing them down. Krystie had grown just under six whole inches in a matter of months, and gained weight! It had crept up on us without us hardly noticing. The massage of her cerebellum area must have taken effect. I spoke to Dr Ali about it, and he said that it was likely that the hypothalamus had been stimulated and resulted in the growth. I couldn't believe it. Needless to say, when I had to buy her new school uniform to begin year 8 of the new school term Krystie needed age 11 school trousers – what a change to the previous year when I had bought her age 7! What a remarkable amount of growth. She looked much better for it, and more mature.

The one drawback with her growth and weight gain was that she had more of herself to move around. Krystie found that she felt tired, and that even with her walking frame she just didn't seem to have the same stamina. I had noticed it too.

As I explained earlier, when we went shopping together, Krystie would not take her walking frame, and didn't like using her wheelchair either. So she used to link arms with me and I would take her weight as she walked. Her recent growth spurt meant that she was a real strain for me now. And because her balance was getting worse, she was relying on me to practically carry her along. I remember one Saturday morning walking in the town centre with her. She felt like a dead weight, and then she lost her balance. I nearly went over with her, and realised that if I had lost my balance too that I would have landed on top of her. What damage would I have caused? It doesn't bear thinking about. So it came to the point where I had to make her use her wheelchair. She felt that I was being overprotective. I felt cruel but I didn't have any other choice. So it was that she started to use a wheelchair at school. Jane Sellar arranged for Krystie to have a manual chair so that she could propel herself, and as a compromise with Krystie agreed that she could use her walking frame during the mornings and the wheelchair during the afternoons. This presented a whole host of new problems. When Krystie walked with her frame, although it was large and bright, she felt that she was up on her feet and was on the same level with her peers. The very nature of a walking frame also creates a protective space around the person using it, and creates a barrier. This helped stop children knocking into her, and they very naturally gave Krystie a wide berth. The chair was quite a different matter. Krystie found herself operating at a lower level. She is always at seat height. The chair doesn't provide the protective bubble around someone, as it were, because you are sat in it. Children could bump right into her; mischievous boys could even grab hold of the handles and push her. It was also quite tiring for Krystie. A manual wheelchair means that you have to propel the wheels yourself. Friedreich's Ataxia means that your muscles are weak and lack power. Negotiating busy corridors and trying to dodge children who don't even see you was taking its toll. To make matters worse, if she did misjudge the direction of her chair sometimes and accidentally roll into people, they were not amused. Krystie found that people moaned at her. I would tell her that she really needed to look very carefully when moving around, but she felt that people didn't look out for her either. Sometimes she felt that people actually did see her, but tried to get in front of her very quickly or squeeze by in small spaces through impatience and then blame her if they got hurt! We had a few tears over these incidents. However, I have to say that I think that the real problem was Krystie accepting that she needed to use her wheelchair more. In her head, she was Krystie, the girl who did not need a wheelchair and could get by. She said that the minute people saw her in the chair they talked differently to her or at times didn't even see her at all.

Things didn't get any better, because Jane had been liaising with the school and been made aware that Krystie was getting very tired. She came to visit us, and recommended that Krystie should be measured to take delivery of an electric wheelchair. She explained that everyone was concerned that Krystie was using too much of her precious energy in simply moving around, and that if she could save some of this energy by using a powered chair she would have more energy left over for learning. Krystie wasn't overjoyed at the prospect but understood that the chair would take several weeks or even months to arrive, and so she agreed to be measured up. In her head I think that she dealt with it by thinking that it was something she could deal with later.

Maybe it was hormones, maybe it was her age (12, just pre-teen), maybe it was just the seemingly rapid changes that were occurring, but whatever it was, Krystie seemed to lose a little bit of her sparkle. I tried to get her to talk openly to me about her feelings, and kept trying to encourage her but she would only tell me so much. She reminded me so much of myself when I was a child. I used to bottle things up inside. I knew that my mom loved me, and would always help if I asked her, but I just felt that I needed to sort things out for myself. I was very self-reliant and so was Krystie. She knew I was there for her, but she needed space to sort things out for herself. I noticed that she started to draw again. Pencil control does not come easily to Krystie, and the effort involved can make her hands tired. She had stopped drawing and painting for a time, because she felt that her art was getting worse not better, but she started to try drawing again. She also wrote poetry and stories. She made things out of paper and glue, really lovely models. I don't really know how she managed to do it, but she did. She became quite insular, and spent a lot of time in her room engaged in these activities. I passed on information to her about wheelchair sports, but she was having none of it. The only physical things that she liked to do were swimming and riding her bike. Incredibly, she could still ride her bike very well. So she did spend some time out in the garden riding her bike; she really enjoyed that she felt free. She liked watching musicals on the television, particularly *The Sound of Music*. She loved it, and knew every line of the film. She thought that Julie Andrews was fantastic, and became a really big fan of hers.

One day I was reading through the newspaper, when I came across a small advertisement. It was in a small box, and had BBC written very boldly at the top. It said:

> BBC2 is researching a programme exploring life-changing moments for disabled people. If you, your child, or someone you know has a disability and is about to embark on some form of life change please call Victoria on . . .

I read and reread the advert. I thought about Krystie's reaction to the *This Morning* programme. She had really loved being involved in the bedroom makeover. When she can talk to people she becomes animated, and particularly enjoys talking to adults. I decided to show her the paper.

A smile crept over her face as she read it and she started to giggle, 'What? Do you think that I should do it?' I nodded. 'They won't be interested in me though will they? Surely not?' I said that I thought that they would be, but that she needed to think about it, because this would be about her. She started to laugh, and was excited by the idea of being involved with television people again. 'Yes,' she said, 'Call them, people should know what goes on in people's lives, perhaps if they saw me, they wouldn't think I was dumb!' So that was that then. I made the call.

Media girl

9

I spoke with Victoria (the girl in the advertisement) who was very friendly. She asked me lots of questions about Krystie and her illness. She explained that she was a researcher working in a team that was making a programme for a BBC documentary series called 'What's Your Problem?' She said that she would have to discuss Krystie's story with the producer, and would get back to me. We spoke a few days' later when she arranged to come and visit us at home. Krystie was bursting with excitement; she couldn't wait. When Victoria arrived, she spoke with Krystie, and they got on really well. Krystie really came into her own; she was full of personality and very chatty. Victoria had brought a small camcorder with her and she filmed Krystie talking. She came to talk to me too, and asked me if I understood the implications, that is that her team would be following us on agreed filming days in order to capture enough film to produce a real fly-on-the-wall type documentary. I explained that we had had a small taster with the bedroom makeover experience, and that Krystie had really enjoyed it. She left and said that the whole team were in the process of meeting people and that they would be back in touch shortly.

A few days later we got another call to say that the producer would like to come and meet Krystie, so we agreed a date. Krystie was like a cat on hot bricks.

The producer came to meet us with Victoria, and she was lovely. Her name was Min Clough. She got on so well with Krystie, and had a lovely way about her. She was unassuming, very down to earth and quite jolly. I got on with her too. She explained that she was making a programme about people who were going through a dramatic life change, and because Krystie was constantly living with change felt that she would be a good subject. The documentary was going to be about three different people, and Krystie was to be one of them. So began a busy spring and summer. The team followed us over a period of approximately three months.

Mitchell thought that we were mad. He didn't particularly mind Krystie being involved in the programme if that was what she wanted to do, just as long as he could be in the background. We were under strict instructions to tell the film crew that he didn't mind being in the background but that he did not want to be interviewed or be highly visible. Nicholas and Anthony were not really bothered, they didn't mind being around; as long as Krystie was quite comfortable they were happy. Harrison and McKenna were 4 and 2 respectively, and confident children, not much trouble at all. It all went over their heads. They were the youngest and so had plenty of attention from everyone. They were quite secure children, and played well together. McKenna was a strong little girl walking and running around. She was so strong that she rarely used her pushchair. So my gamble had paid off. It seemed that I would never have to cope with the difficult scenario of using a pushchair and wheelchair at the same time.

Krystie was filmed in her bedroom, in the swimming pool, in the garden, on her bike and at school. The crew were able to capture the fact that she was indeed living through momentous change. It was quite a contrast to watch the opening shots of her riding her bike, and then to see her using her wheelchair at school. The team filmed us in London visiting Dr Ali and watched her having a massage. Min talked to Krystie on camera quite a lot about how she felt about the changes that she was going through. Krystie came across as a very mature and thoughtful young lady. She was so optimistic. I think that making that programme was really quite therapeutic for her because it gave her the platform to show the world that she was 'normal'.

Min also interviewed me. I wanted to be quite open about how I felt, and so I talked about the various treatments that we pursued to try and help keep Krystie on her feet. I hoped that people would see me for what I was, a mother trying to do her best under the circumstances.

During one of her chats with Krystie, Min found out about her art, and her disappointment in her diminishing abilities. Min agreed with me that actually it was Krystie's attitude to the situation that was causing the problem. So I arranged to take her to the Tate Gallery in London so that she could look at the work of the great painter Vincent Van Gogh. She enjoyed the day, but was still quite adamant that she preferred more precise drawing techniques!

Thomas Telford were very helpful in agreeing to allow the BBC to film Krystie at school. Having a film crew follow you around gave Krystie certain notoriety and helped her to feel a bit special. She stopped feeling like the underdog and her true personality began to blossom.

Thomas Telford is a school that celebrates achievement, and once a year they arrange a special awards evening. It is an invitation-only event. The teachers nominate children for various awards and no one actually knows anything about it until the invitation arrives on the doormat by post. We received such an invite for Krystie. You have no idea which award your child will receive. The school presents awards for academic, sporting, musical and dramatic achievements. In addition they also give personality and general achievement awards. Krystie could not believe it; she had recently commented that she felt like she never shone at anything. A number of her friends were performing well at sports or in drama. Lots of pupils were performing exceptionally well academically, so I think that Krystie felt that she couldn't compete at any level. She could not imagine what award she could possibly be given.

We went along to the evening and sat proudly with the other parents. It was an uplifting evening to hear about so many young people who were being recognised for their varying achievements. Finally the headmaster announced the special awards categories. He gave out one award, which was duly accepted by the successful young person. As the applause died down, he continued with his next award speech. The words that he was saying were beautiful, and then I realised that he was talking about Krystie; I could not stop the tears. The award was the Emma Shaw Personality of the Year Award and the citation was:

> The award goes to a very special young lady who has also managed to overcome her difficulties in order to make the most of school life. She goes about her business every day with a beaming smile and a chirpy disposition that rubs off on everyone around her. She has even charmed her way on to television, when she managed a team of designers in remodelling her

room. Needless to say she made sure they stuck to the brief she set.

Krystie the rest of the students in school will be thrilled for you and I know Mr and Mrs Shaw will be very pleased to hear you have received the Emma Shaw Personality of the Year Award.

What a lovely award. Krystie went up to collect it. She was radiant. She was awarded a crystal clock as a memento, and of course her name would be engraved on the school's trophy. It was the affirmation that she needed that people still valued her in spite of her challenges. In his speech, the headmaster had spoken about Krystie's cheerfulness, and the effect this had on other people. It made me realise that she must have been more serious at home because of the efforts that she was making at school – the daily face that she presented to the world. She obviously covered her insecurities well. The presentation took place just before the summer holidays, so it was the perfect end to her first academic year at Thomas Telford.

Krystie

Oh yes, Personality of the Year, my first year at Thomas Telford and I got an award! Apart from being rather bemused and confused by the whole idea of an 'Achievement Evening' I felt rather honoured. I understood the award to be in memory of a student who unfortunately died a few years before I first went to the school.

Going up to collect the trophy felt unbelievable, I'd never been good at sports or anything, and so had never really had the opportunity to get anything like a trophy or medal. As I stood there in front of the camera shaking the hand of a dignitary, I couldn't help but wonder what was so special about me?

In October it was time for the documentary that she had been involved in to be screened. It was entitled *Free Wheelers*. We only got a chance to watch it the day before it went out, so it was too late to change anything even if we did have any complaints. Fortunately we didn't.

Considering how much time that the team had spent with us, it was surprising how much of the filming that they captured had ended up on the cutting-room floor. I felt that the finished programme had missed out a lot of the lighter happier times, and focused on the heavier, perhaps less cheerful moments. However, I could also appreciate that Min was trying to capture in a very short space of time Krystie's gut reaction to the changes that she was living through. Krystie being a child was brutally honest, she wasn't interested in being politically correct, so she said what she felt. I sat and watched the programme on the evening that it went out with the rest of the family and was nervous about the reception that it would get. *The Times* had listed it as 'the one to watch', and printed a nice picture of Krystie, but the public reception would be the test.

Krystie

Free Wheelers, yes the second time I was on tele. Filming was absolutely, spectacularly, fantabulously exciting. Min the producer is really nice, and even now we remain friends. But afterwards, I was recognised on the street, which was insane! I was in ASDA one day when someone grabbed my shoulders as I innocently looked at the cheese stand. Immediately I spun round. 'I saw you on tele,' a complete stranger said excitedly. Although I found it weird I gotta say I loved the buzz I got, like a celebrity gets I expect.

The programme got a fantastic reaction. The BBC website got lots of emails; lots of people contacted us. I was surprised at the number of people in our area that stopped us to say that they had enjoyed watching Krystie on television. Not all the feedback was positive though, and I have to say that the obvious strength of emotion and feeling in some people's views was quite unnerving. It seemed that the politically correct brigade were not altogether happy with Krystie's candour and mine. Quite a few emails were directed at me personally, asking what kind of mother was I to keep forcing my child up on her feet, when I could have let her use a wheelchair. The comment around those emails flew backwards and forwards. So I sent an email response in, and reminded the audience that they saw twenty minutes of film out of three months' worth. Furthermore,

Krystie and I were not party to the editing of the film. Whilst I could understand their view, they needed to appreciate that Krystie herself wanted to maintain her ability to walk, and I was simply helping her to do that. However, we were quite happy to use a wheelchair full-time when Krystie felt that it was the right time to do that. My email more or less closed down the negative backlash, and I even received an apology.

Jane Sellar was not happy either. Towards the end of the film, Krystie had answered a question by stating words to the effect that I was busy with work and the little ones and so she didn't always talk to me. Jane could not believe that Min had put that in the film because she said that she knew that I talked to Krystie all the time. I admitted that I had felt a little sensitive about that, too, but I felt that Min had to portray what she wanted to. I also knew that Krystie meant something slightly different to what actually came out of her mouth. I was secure in the knowledge that Krystie could talk to me whenever she wanted to, and so was Krystie. But I also knew that she was a little bit like me in that she chose to keep a lot of what she felt to herself because she knew that there are no answers to some things. I decided that it didn't matter what I thought about the programme, it mattered what Krystie thought. I trusted Min, and I knew that she made that programme with the greatest integrity. We can all of us worry too much about what other people think, the only thing that mattered in this was Krystie. So I wasn't upset.

I had let the Ataxia society know about the programme, and they had let their members know about it so that they could watch the programme if they wanted too. Once the programme had been screened, the *Daily Mail* ran a full-page story on Krystie, and some magazines did too. I requested that these give the details of Ataxia UK to enable people to make donations for research, which they did.

Lots of people wrote letters to Min asking her to pass them on to Krystie. Some of these were very touching. I couldn't quite believe that people took the time to write. She had made such a big impression on them. Some wrote about how they had been depressed, but watching Krystie had made them realise that they had nothing to be depressed about. Others wrote saying that she should be on television since she had talked more sense than a lot of grown-ups. Krystie couldn't believe the reaction. Some people even sent her money. It was a reminder that there are lots of good people on this earth, it really was. Krystie was also interviewed on local radio, and appeared on our regional teatime news. She loved it all! She handled it all well, and took it all in her stride (so to speak!). I call her my media girl.

The highs and lows of 2004 10

After all the previous excitement I don't know how we got back to normal really. The year had flown by; before we knew it we had started 2003.

A lady called Louise Dyson who runs an agency for disabled models and actors called VisABLE People contacted us, asking if she could sign Krystie to her books. She had watched Krystie in *Free Wheelers* and thought that she came across very well. She had tracked us down via the BBC. She put her forward for a part in the children's series called *Tracy Beaker*. Unfortunately Krystie didn't get the part, but she loved auditioning for it and it opened a new world of possibilities for her. She started to think about what career she could pursue when she eventually left school and for the first time considered acting.

Krystie started to write; she wrote some really good stories. Her creativity seemed to be diverted away from art and into writing. She said that she either wanted to work in television or write, and so began to develop her craft.

It was a quiet year really. Krystie took delivery of her electric chair, which she wasn't that ecstatic about. The professional opinion was that she should use the chair for school, to conserve energy. She had had time to get used to the idea so she agreed to use it, but she found the change difficult. She much preferred her manual wheelchair, so we got into the routine of using the manual chair out of school, and the electric chair at school. The one thing that she did find amusing about the electric chair was that she had to take a 'driving test'. A nice gentleman from wheelchair services came out to see us, and took us out for a road test. Actually I had to be tested steering the chair whilst Krystie was sitting in it too (which was hilarious). The chair has a button on the back that allows you to divert the controls from the user to an assistant who can push from the back. I kept confusing my left and right. Eventually I got to grips with the controls but Krystie said that she didn't feel safe with me being in the driving seat! Krystie on the other hand was excellent. She manoeuvred it very well indeed; she found the whole episode highly amusing. As the gentleman reminded us, though, it was a serious matter because the chair weighed approx half a ton and was capable of causing serious damage. We joked about putting Krystie in control of a potentially dangerous weapon, she smiled wickedly and said that she could think of a few people that she wouldn't mind 'clipping'!

A school trip came up for London. It was a theatre trip, and the children were going to stay overnight in a hotel. Krystie like her classmates was keen to go, and so put her name down on the 'yes, interested' list. She was told that she would only be able to go if she was accompanied. She was not happy. When you are 13 and trying to fit in and be cool, the last thing that you want to do is take your mom on a school trip. I had a conversation with the teachers, and said that I wasn't happy about their decision either. However, they explained that since this was an extra-curricular trip that they could not supply an assistant. All the teachers who were travelling preferred to have someone else travel with Krystie; I guess that they found her condition daunting. What could I say? I could understand their point of view, but I could also understand Krystie's. So we arrived at a compromise. I arranged for an adult to accompany her, and the school was happy because Krystie was not travelling alone. When Krystie was younger, a family friend had looked after her for me when I worked part-time and Krystie was really fond of her younger sister, Demelza. She was in her early twenties now, so responsible but really 'cool' too. She loved Krystie and when she grew up herself had looked after Krystie for me from time to time. I approached her, and she agreed to help out. She got on well with everyone; was great fun and more importantly Krystie didn't lose face with her friends.

* * *

Meanwhile, my older son Nicholas had met a girl called Stephanie, and after going out together for a couple of years had set a date for their wedding. It was to take place in September 2003. Krystie and McKenna were going to be bridesmaids along with Steph's two sisters. Krystie was adamant that she was going to walk down the aisle. At this stage Krystie could walk a little but really needed support or someone to lean on. The only way that I could see her managing was if someone helped her. The most practical solution was to ask Anthony to escort her down the aisle, which he agreed to do straight away. Krystie moaned about the fact that she would have to use her wheelchair at the wedding reception. She felt that it was bulky and ugly. Mitch and I agreed to find her a 'nifty' machine. We looked at brochures and found her a sporty lightweight sports chair made by Küschall. It was fantastic. When Krystie sat in the chair you still saw her. It was so unobtrusive and it looked really cool. At £1,800 it wasn't cheap, but we knew that it would make a big difference to her self-image. So we ordered one for her. It arrived two days before the wedding. She was over the moon.

The day arrived; it was hot and sunny. Krystie wore a long lilac dress and had her hair put up. She looked beautiful. I will never forget her beaming face as she walked smoothly and steadily down the aisle that day. No jerky movements, and no stumbling. Anthony says that he took a lot of her weight but my goodness her grit and determination certainly kicked into place. I was always bound to cry: my eldest son, my firstborn, was getting married, but Krystie's walk down the aisle added a poignancy to the occasion. I just knew that I would probably never ever see her make such a walk again. She knew it too. She used her new 'groovy chair' at the reception and looked really happy and settled. The whole day was beautiful and everyone enjoyed it.

However, in December, Harrison and McKenna caught chicken pox. They weren't too poorly with it, but it's not a pleasant illness. Being the generous souls that they are they passed it on to Krystie, who had avoided catching it off Nicholas and Anthony several years earlier.

She was 13 now, so late to have the virus compared to a lot of children. She got a bad dose of it and really suffered. She took to her bed, absolutely covered in spots. Her face was badly affected, and we were both worried about the scars. Up until this point Krystie had a very clear unmarked complexion, but we could tell that these spots were going to leave marks. After two weeks of the virus I expected her to start to recover, but she didn't. I gave her the usual medicines for children, and plenty of hot drinks and light food (if she would eat it), but she just seemed to get worse. Three weeks into the illness, I thought that a proper bath might help her to feel better, because I had been washing her in her bed. I helped her to the bathroom and ran the bath. I helped her get into the water, turned round to get something and when I turned back to look at her I was completely shocked to find that she was slipping under the water. I am not sure whether it was the heat or just weakness but she was disappearing under water. I dived to grab her, but really struggled to pull her up. She was slipping under again. I grabbed the plug so that the water would start to empty, and shouted for Anthony, who happened to be home. She was like a floppy rag doll, and could not help herself. I somehow managed to get her out of the bath even though she was lying down. Once on the bathroom floor, she was just too weak to hold herself up. Anthony appeared, and I asked him to carry her downstairs for me. He had to carry her like you would carry a baby or a young child. I felt very shook up, and upset. I got her dried off and back into bed, where she fell asleep. I left her to rest for about an hour and then went back to check on her. She was still asleep. I wanted her to eat or drink something, so I shook her gently, and as she responded I could see that she was really quite dopey. I felt really worried by now, and went to telephone the surgery to request that the doctor come out to see her. He arrived about half an hour later. He listened to me, and examined her. You should have called me days ago he said. The virus is attacking her heart and lungs, I am going to give her some very strong anti-virus drugs, but if she is not any better in the next few hours, she will have to go into hospital. I felt really bad, as if I had let her down. But I thought that she 'just' had chicken pox like the other children, and that it was maybe going to take her longer to get over it. Fortunately the drugs worked very quickly indeed; by the next day she was sitting up in bed. When I saw Dr Anderson a few weeks later and told her about the incident, she explained that chicken pox can attack the cerebellum area of the brain and that was why it could have had such a profound effect on Krystie. She got terrible scars, especially on her face. She couldn't believe it. I can remember her looking into a mirror and saying, 'Oh great, not only am I sat in this wheelchair, but now my face looks terrible.' My sister-in-law Claudine brought her some pure vitamin E oil. We both encouraged her to use it explaining that it might help her skin to heal. I also told her that the marks would fade over time. I must admit that I was upset about the marks too. Krystie's complexion had been so smooth and unblemished, now it was covered with really dark chicken pox marks that were really, really noticeable. At 13, it's not what you want is it? I prayed that the oil and time would fade them out. Looking at her now, they have faded; she does have slight marks but they are nothing like they were. I am sure that they will continue to fade even more over the next few years. Even though she recovered, she lost a lot of strength in her legs and has never recovered the abilities that she had prior to catching chicken pox. That virus finally closed the door on her being able to walk even a couple of steps. Up until this point, she had been able to walk a little, especially if she held on to something or someone; not anymore, she couldn't even take her own weight. Krystie couldn't believe it. I couldn't help but remember the wedding just a few weeks earlier; how quickly things change. We took a call from the hospital at this time, to say that Dr Anderson wanted Krystie to get a flu jab as soon as possible because she felt that her body had taken enough. It was all a reminder to me that her system is very delicate, and that you cannot afford to be complacent with her.

Another year ended and so began 2004. Krystie was still weak from the chicken pox. It was a good job that she had begun using her electric wheelchair because she really didn't have the strength to propel her manual one all day. She was even using her electric chair at home now! She really didn't like her electric chair. It was very big compared to a manual chair, and Krystie felt that people treated her differently once she was in it. She says that people are a bit odd once they see you in a manual chair, but that their reaction to an electric chair is even worse. She felt so much weaker after having chicken pox and knowing this upset her. She asked me if she would ever recover her strength. I felt that she probably would. We had noticed a pattern in that she would catch a bug, which would seem to devastate her system and take a little bit more of her muscle control, and then over the course of a few weeks she would recover some of the strength that she had lost. I have to say that she never got it all back, but she did recover some.

Krystie was 14 in the March and became very self-conscious. She wanted to look and feel like a normal teenager. She was obviously noticing boys, but felt that she was completely invisible to them. She hated looking different, and was very aware of her limitations. She really started to voice her irritation at the equipment that people wanted her to use. One example particularly springs to mind. The teachers and the medics had suggested that she use a tray on her wheelchair so that she could get over the problem of being at an awkward height for desks. A tray was delivered to us and fitted to her chair. She was indignant and upset. She refused to use it. In between tears she asked me why we were trying to make her look like 'a div' (her words!). She said that people already thought that she was odd, and with a tray on her chair she would look like a granny! She would not have it. I just cannot find it within myself to force her to use these things. I think that she has enough to put up with so I will not force her to do things that she really doesn't want to do. I remember being a teenager at school (it wasn't that long ago!), and I know how important it is to feel confident about yourself. Her body image was at an all-time low. She felt that everyone around her had boyfriends, or people queuing up to ask them out; but she had no one. She really felt it, and was not about to do anything else that she felt made her look even more odd. I said that she should do what she felt most comfortable doing; if she was happy, then so was I.

Around this time Krystie, decided that she didn't really want to pursue any more alternative treatments. We argued about it, but she really felt that she had had enough. In the end, I felt that she needed to do what she felt was right. Krystie is not stupid, she can read information and understand it; I felt that she had the right to make some decisions about her body. So we stopped the massage, and any supplements.

Krystie

Alternative treatments, I remember those definitely — don't think I'll ever forget them. I don't really have much to say on the matter, except that they both hurt, teehee. But I've gotta say they kept me walking for a long time. I've been thinking about going back for them again actually because although I didn't realise it at the time, they did help slow down the progress of my Friedreich's. I would definitely recommend both Basil and Dr Ali; they were very nice, although they did hurt!

I looked for ways to help Krystie be more social, because it can be quite restrictive in her chair. I told her about wheelchair basketball, and riding for the disabled, but she wasn't interested. I think that her head hadn't caught up with her body. Yes, she used her wheelchair, and yes, she knows her limitations, but in her head she's still the 9-year-old

Krystie who can walk. It worried me, but what could I do? I figured that she would eventually come to terms with everything, I would just have to wait.

The year ticked along without too much excitement. Krystie had all her usual annual checks. In July it was time for her spinal check. In 2003, the doctors had said that her spine was showing a slight curvature (scoliosis) but that it wasn't too bad. We arrived at the hospital expecting a similar explanation this time too. I knew that scoliosis is a common complaint amongst FA sufferers, but her back looked fine to me. She had some X-rays and then we went in to see the doctor. He was looking at them. He explained that actually her spine had moved almost a degree every single month since her last appointment. In medical terms, that was quite a rapid progression. He explained that we needed to rectify the curvature as soon as possible, because if we didn't the spine would curve over too much and eventually this would crush her heart and her lungs. She already had cardiomyopathy, so we needed to make sure that we didn't add pressure to the heart. The risks were spelled out to us. If we left the spine, it would continue to curve, and eventually put too much pressure on her heart and lungs which would be painful and dangerous. In addition, her heart would need to be assessed to understand the risks to her during surgery. This particular surgeon was recommending a full-length spinal fusion, meaning that it would be a long operation with very heavy blood loss. The heavy blood loss combined with a weak heart was a potentially fatal combination. As if that were not enough there was the additional risk of paralysis. Krystie's eyes grew wider with each statement that the doctor made. 'So am I at risk of being paralysed then?' she asked. He looked at her and said, 'If you lose a lot of blood and we can't replace it you are more at risk of not waking up.' Krystie simply said OK and nodded. The doctor looked at me and continued, 'Mrs Maddox, you are between a rock and a hard place, you are damned if you do and damned if you don't.' For once I was completely shocked. I knew scoliosis was a common complaint with FA, but I had not seen this coming; her back looked fine to me. I didn't quite know what to do. We left saying that we needed time to think. The doctor reminded me that with Krystie's heart condition, which could deteriorate at any time, we would be wiser to act quickly. We started the hour's drive home, and Krystie, who was understandably worried, started to ask me questions. As usual I answered them honestly and tactfully. I always look for the positive slant, and let her know that I am there to help her and stand by her. But in the cold light of day, in the case of such an illness, it doesn't seem enough. I cannot take the worry or pain away. The effects and consequences of anything are experienced directly by Krystie. She must face the stark reality of everything and feel it all. I often feel like I am using the dregs from a bucket to put out a forest fire. I can never do enough. I can never take the reality and harshness away.

Once I could be on my own I was devastated. For the first time since her diagnosis her mortality was staring me right in the face. I felt sick. I could not imagine Krystie not being around. The risks were very real, and of course you could push them out of your mind and think only positive thoughts but that didn't remove them, it simply covered them over.

We had started a nail bar six months before McKenna was born (I know, as if we didn't have enough on our plates!). Now, I just felt like I had too much. I had a family, the consultancy, the nail bar and Krystie. Something had to give. We decided to close the nail bar. It was sad to have to do this, but I could not do everything any more. I felt like I had a crushing weight on my shoulders and I had to make my life 'seem' simpler. Our staff had been with us for four years and were like family. I managed to find a hair salon within the town centre that was prepared to buy the goodwill and stock from the business and also take on the staff, and so effectively transfer the business to their premises. I felt that we had done our best for the girls, at least they all kept jobs.

Just a few weeks later a letter from Thomas Telford arrived; it was an invitation to the 2004 achievement evening. Krystie had been nominated again; she could not believe it. We attended the evening with my mother and waited to see what award she would receive. It was the Victoria Harper Celebration Award for Achievement. The citation was:

> Krystie is a student who will not let her physical challenges be a barrier to her school or social life. This student insisted on doing her SATs just like the rest of her year group, even though she could have justifiably opted out, and insisted on handwriting her work, which is quite a feat. She made amazing gains in all three subjects; most notably Maths, which she confesses, is not her favourite subject. When the opportunity came to go on a theatre trip to London with the English Department, she joined the whistle-stop sightseeing tour and theatre visits with more

energy than most which just goes to show that where there is a will there is a way.

I couldn't help it, I cried with pride, but I also cried with fear. I caught myself wondering if this was to be her last few months alive. She was so full of life, such a vibrant character, it just didn't make sense. At times there does not seem to be a good enough answer for anything. There is no one, absolutely no one, who can help you. At such times people often find comfort in faith. Faith had played a big part in my life for many years; now more than at any other time I found myself seriously contemplating the question: well, what about faith?

What about faith? 11

My mother had become a Jehovah's Witness when I was a child. She didn't make a quick decision; it had taken her some time to finally be baptised in the faith. Actually my earliest recollection of my mom and the Jehovah's Witnesses was her shouting at them as they stood on our doorstep! She was shouting at them because her brother had 'joined' the faith, and she was not at all happy about it. But one day when someone else knocked at her door, they asked her a question that made her think. Mom had always been a Catholic. She had been christened when she was a child. My grandfather was from Liverpool and he was a staunch Catholic, insisting that his children were christened and brought up in his church rather than my grandmother's, which was Church of England. Like a lot of people they had a belief in God, but church attendance was reserved for high days and holidays (if at all).

For whatever reason, on this particular day, the question that had just been put to my mother made her think. She talked with the strangers on her doorstep, and for once didn't send them away with a flea in their ear. She accepted the magazines that they were offering, the *Watchtower* and *Awake*, and said that they could call again. They visited her several times, and mom had more and more questions which they always answered direct from the Bible. She eventually started to study the Bible with them and became quite interested. I was 6 at the time, a typical nosey little girl, who wanted to be in on everything. So I made sure that I was always around to listen when they called; I really enjoyed listening to them. I was a bright child who could read really well, and so when they offered me a children's book I accepted it and read the lot. I read it over and over again. The Bible is at one level a very simple collection of stories, but the morals or meaning of those stories are powerful. I really began to develop my own faith. Mom decided that she wasn't really ready to commit to the religion after all, and so started to miss her Bible studies, and eventually stopped them altogether. Just a few months later we all became poorly with the measles and Andrew died.

Mom decided that she wanted the Witnesses to give a Bible-based talk at the funeral, which they did. Once the funeral was over she didn't go back to the meetings or study, mentally she just wasn't up to it. I do remember that she spent a lot of time reading the Bible though. I guess that she was looking for answers and comfort. The King James Version of the Bible was to hand, always on the arm of her chair.

I missed the ladies coming to talk about the Bible, and made sure that every book and every magazine that they had ever left with us was in my bedroom. I also had the New World Translation of the Bible; I treated all those publications like gold. I would read them daily and for hours. I enjoyed learning about the Bible. A lot of the books were talking about its prophecies, explaining what they meant; I found it all fascinating.

I have found that most people consider the Witnesses to be a strange religion. You can announce that you are Catholic, Church of England, or Methodist and no one bats an eye – but tell them you are a Jehovah's Witness and they run a mile! Like most prejudices these reactions stem from ignorance and misunderstanding.

Jehovah's Witnesses on the whole are good people. It's like every-thing in life: no matter what colour or race, no matter what religion or organisation, there are good and bad people in everything. In my expe-rience the vast majority of Witnesses are good, genuine, law-abiding people who are just trying to live their lives in accordance with the Bible. It has to be said that if we all followed the basic principles recorded in that book like those captured in the Ten Commandments then we wouldn't have half the trouble in the world that exists today. Jesus took the law a step further, when he said that actually he was going to replace the Ten Commandments with just two: love God with your whole heart and love your neighbour as yourself. So simple, because if we all loved our neighbours as much as we love ourselves, then we would never do anything to hurt anybody, and if we truly loved God then we would do our level best to follow his guidance. That's what appealed to me, the simple common sense of it all.

After my mother had given birth to Sonia, my youngest sister, she says that she was looking at her sleeping peacefully one day and she suddenly asked herself why she had had another baby. She remembers thinking, if this child doesn't die today, tomorrow or next year then she will die eventually, we all do. So what is the point of life? She pondered the question and felt that the only people who had ever come close to satisfying it were the Witnesses, and they had answered it direct from the Bible. So to my surprise, and pleasure, she announced that we would be going back to the meetings and making some time in our lives for faith. I was 10 years old.

I was so happy. I had always wanted to go back to the meetings, and had asked my mother to take me many times over the years. The religion is quite structured and means that you have to spend time actually reading and studying the Bible for yourself. The meetings are scheduled with three during the week and two on a Sunday. You really need to keep up with the personal Bible study because the information that you learn is covered at the meetings. The study schedule is distributed monthly in advance. So the subjects that are covered and discussed are the same all around the country. Usually you would attend an hour-long meeting on a Tuesday evening, where you study the basic teachings of the Bible. Followed by two one-hour meetings that run one after the other on a Thursday evening. The first meeting is a school where you register to give Bible-based talks, which are critiqued by an older man in the congregation. The purpose of the school is to develop your ability to speak in public and reason with people. It provides excellent training. The second hour is to talk about various Bible topics; it is usually interactive, so people from the audience can comment; and it often uses people to give demonstrations by role-play. The Sunday meeting runs for two hours, the first hour is a Bible-based sermon, and the second hour is a question and answer study of the *Watchtower*. I always enjoyed the meetings, but then I love reading and learning. I also found the congregation to be supportive and friendly. My teenage years were immersed in the congregation. I made good friends and met my first husband there. Having a strong faith does give you a contentment and inner peace. It also gives you a purpose. When I was growing up it provided good guidelines and I always felt that it kept me out of trouble. I can remember thinking that even when my parents were not around that God was probably watching! Do you know what? I don't think that was a bad attitude to have at all.

I married in the faith, and had my children in the faith. I explained earlier that it was my depression after having Krystie that changed everything, when I became ill and fell apart. I couldn't run our home properly at that time let alone fit everything else in. My husband was trying his best to be a strong 'Brother' in the congregation and so was often busy, out on ministerial duties. As I said at the beginning of this story, he could not understand what had happened to his very capable wife. I, on the other hand, could not forgive him for not noticing how I was feeling, and how ill I was. I felt that I was being left alone to cope. Our marriage, as you know, eventually broke down.

It came as a great shock to everyone – family, friends, the congregation. We had been such a strong family unit; no one could understand what had gone wrong. You can't explain it; all I can say is that when you have led such a Bible-coded life, that you don't walk away from your marriage lightly. Even though it was hard, it was the right thing to do, but that doesn't stop you feeling guilty. Our lives changed drastically after the divorce. I kept the children with me, and took on the full responsibility of caring for them. I really was on my own now and had to work really hard to make sure that the impact on the children was minimised.

After any divorce most people say that friendships change, and people back away. I found that to be the case with the congregation. However, you can't be sure that your perception is right because it could be your own insecurities or conscience that makes you react differently to things. I still believed the Bible, and still found faith a strengthening aid, but you are keenly aware that you have very badly missed the target.

Once I met Mitchell, who is not a Jehovah's Witness, it seemed as though I had created another stumbling block in my attempt to recover my close standing with God, because the Bible encourages you to 'marry only in the Lord'. I know that every religion will apply that scripture to their own particular faith, but it makes sense whatever religion you are. If you have decided to make religion central to your life and intend to practise that faith, why marry someone who does not share the same view? You will not agree on the basics, and you have the potential to cause an additional pressure point in your relationship. However, it's very difficult to think that clearly about things when you have been suffering with post-natal depression, have just got divorced and feel quite alone. When I met Mitchell he was one of the few people who was truly supportive. Then when you get to know someone, and fall in love, your heart takes over and it has a very strong pull indeed.

Mitchell was more disturbed about me being a Jehovah's Witness than the fact that I had three children and was divorced! But working with me, he got to see that I was harmless. Talking to me, he came to realise that I was a rational person, who thought about things. He had all the usual questions about those 'mad, door-knocking nuisance people'. I answered them, and showed him the Scriptures from the Bible that explained why we do and believe certain things. He could see that I genuinely believed the Bible, and that I used the Bible to guide my life. He said that he would never want to become a Jehovah's Witness himself but he thought that they were decent people. He had been friends with a lad whose mother was a Witness when he was at school, so had known other Witnesses before me. He also said that he didn't mind me sticking to what I believed in. He didn't have a problem with it at all. So because we got on so well, and because he was also really good with my children, and because I fell in love with him, we eventually got married. I carried on attending meetings. I still loved reading the literature, and studying the Bible; I maintained my faith. I suppose that I was living in a familiar scenario. My own father had never been a Jehovah's Witness; he never stopped us going along, and didn't really mind our faith. He did sometimes say that he thought that we were mad to go out knocking on doors and to spend so much time at meetings but he also felt that the principles provided a good code to live your life by. They say you end up marrying someone like your father, and in that sense I had, because Mitch is exactly the same.

When Krystie was diagnosed with Friedreich's Ataxia, I was very glad to have a faith because I could pray for strength to cope and I thought a lot about the Bible-based hope for the future. I could also talk to the children about those things and remind Krystie about them too. I have to admit that once I got married and had Harrison I stopped attending all five meetings that took place during the course of a week. I just couldn't maintain that commitment. I was not the same strong person that I had been before I had had Krystie. I was more tired, and could only do so much in a day. Having driven myself so hard in the past to do everything, and ending up at rock-bottom, I just couldn't do it anymore. I knew my limits, and I listened to my body. I tried to attend at least three meetings a week, and sometimes managed four, but it was hard. As time moved on I found myself looking after two babies, managing two teenagers, moving and then doing up a house, working and then supporting Krystie. On top of this I was attending multiple hospital appointments. During the year 2001, which was the 'peak' year for hospital visits, I had appointments every single month (and sometimes every week)! But on top of this I had the two little ones, who also had their own baby clinic appointments and toddler assessments. I was constantly chasing my tail. If I could make two meetings in a week then I had achieved a lot because I was just pushed to the absolute limit. So it would be true to say that I was no longer immersed in the congregation, but just hanging on by my fingertips.

The biggest single fact that most people know about Jehovah's Witnesses is that they do not accept blood transfusions. It is a controversial stance that attracts criticism, though it would be fair to say that it is a view that is becoming more popular amongst a variety of people today. It wasn't something that I ever worried about. I understood why the Witnesses make that stand, and again it's simply because Scriptures in both the Old and New Testament state that blood is sacred to God, and must be poured out on the ground, not taken into the body; a straightforward set of statements. Over the years medical advancements have to a large degree minimised the risk that sticking to those Scriptures bring. I have known many Jehovah's Witnesses who have undergone major surgery without blood and been absolutely fine.

The issue had personally touched me when I suffered from placenta praevia when I was carrying Harrison. I haemorrhaged twice. I didn't have blood transfusions. I accept that my bleeds were not catastrophic, they were small controlled bleeds, however the doctors were worried in case they changed suddenly and became threatening. I didn't feel traumatised. I was concerned about the children, but didn't feel that I should be making any other choice. Both times I was fine.

Surgery is always about risk. Every medical procedure carries a degree of risk. I have had four wisdom teeth removed, a lump taken from by breast and two Caesareans. I also had the infamous piles op! Each time I have requested to sign an instruction that says I do not wish to use blood. Each time the medics involved have been happy to operate under those conditions. The only time that I noted any real concern was when I had placenta praevia, but that turned out fine.

The thing is, blood is peculiar to each individual person. Yes you can group blood types, like you can group apples and pears, but no two bloods are exactly the same. That is why blood samples are used for genetic fingerprinting. Blood samples are accepted as conclusive evidence in court because it is accepted that blood is like a fingerprint and no two bloods are exactly the same. This means that when you do receive blood, although it obviously does serve a purpose in surgery (by expanding the volume of blood in your body and, in severe blood loss, transporting a very small degree of oxygen – definitely not as much as you might think!), it does not work like your own blood does. It does not work to full capacity transporting oxygen. In fact your own body recognises that your body has been given foreign tissue, and actually starts working to reject it. This rejection process can slow down the recovery time post surgery, and it is widely reported that time and time again Jehovah's Witnesses recover very quickly after surgery. Jehovah's Witnesses have successfully been accepting other types of blood expanders for many years now. Blood expanders that are not rejected by the body. Surgeons have also refined their operating techniques, by using different methods. For instance, lowering the body temperature to slow down bleeding, cauterising veins so that they don't bleed, taking extra care to clamp veins quickly and accurately to minimise blood loss and in the last few years using machines like cell savers that simply extend your own circulatory system by attaching to your body, collecting spilled blood, cleaning it and pumping it back into you. All of these advances have been advantageous to all kinds of people, since many doctors who know the risks involved in using real blood choose wherever possible not to use it.

The problem we faced was that in Krystie's case we were told by the scoliosis surgeon that her operation was one of those where he believed that blood was the only thing that would make the difference. That is why he told Krystie that she was more at risk of not waking up if she lost too much blood.

I have to tell you that I felt in complete turmoil. It was one thing to refuse blood for myself, but my child, well that was quite another. If anything was going to make me question my faith it was this situation. The other thing was that since I was not attending all the meetings and was on the outside of the congregation, so to speak, would I still feel the same? I was sure about one thing, the decisions that Krystie and I made over the next few months had to be our own personal decisions not influenced by anyone else. We had to be happy with them.

Krystie said that she preferred not to have blood. We talked about it a lot, and then I told her that she really needed to be sure that she felt strongly about that decision. I told her that she should put every single person out of her mind and think about the Bible, God and herself. She shouldn't even worry about me. I made sure that she had literature that discussed the blood issue to read, and I simply left her to mull everything over. I reminded her that she could also pray about it, and over time she would know what felt right for her. I did the same.

However, for me, there was a query that was disturbing me. You see when I thought back to twenty or so years ago, the blood issue was very straightforward. Jehovah's Witnesses did not accept blood transfusions or blood products. In other words it was a straight yes/no decision. Today the situation is quite different. Medical advancement is such that blood can be broken down into its component parts. So, for example, blood is made up of water, albumin and globulins to name just a few ingredients. Scientists have actually been able to break it down into its tiny component parts. This ability has given Witnesses more options on transfusions, because what they say is that whilst the Bible teachings indicate that you cannot accept whole blood, that each individual can make their own decision as to whether or not they could accept blood components (such as albumin and immune globulins). For example, blood is also made up of water, and we all drink water. At a time when I was stressed and worried about my daughter, I found this information confusing because in my mind it felt like if I put all the allowable components into a test tube and shook them up that surely I would very nearly arrive at blood. Actually this isn't quite the case, because a Witness would never accept the red blood cells themselves, but that's what it felt like. I telephoned the headquarters of the Witnesses both in America and London, and spoke to someone on the helplines. I explained how I felt and they listened and talked to me about the options I had. You must remember that the decisions that any Witnesses make are individual and private, based on their own individual conscience. Some people will choose to take as many component parts as they can, others will tread the middle ground, and others will have absolutely no components at all. I did feel very irritated by all of this, I felt that actually the decision was harder to make. In the end I kept praying about it and took my own advice; I didn't think about anyone else, except Krystie, God, the Bible and myself. I read those simple Scriptures and decided that my faith meant that I would prefer bloodless surgery. I would accept blood expanders, and the allowable component parts if necessary and also the use of the cell-saver machine. However, I felt that the best key to a successful outcome was locating a highly trained surgeon whom I could trust. Krystie felt the same; without my telling her what my feelings were.

So my faith in the Bible remains, I do believe in God, and I do still follow the Witness faith. I am not a steadfast pillar of the congregation, and in fact at this point in time am trying to get some regularity back into my attendance. Mitchell does not mind the little ones coming to meetings with me; his only comment is that they must also know and understand his familys' views on things, and attend some of their family services, which are Church of England. I married Mitchell, and our children are both of ours, so I am not about to argue over his requests. Our children will learn two sides and make their choices when they are old enough to do so. The lesson of getting along together is a valuable one for them to learn I'm sure.

Krystie's illness didn't make me lose my faith in God, and I don't blame him for her condition. The Bible actually explains why these things happen and does talk about a hope for the future and therefore for Krystie. I just think that the daily grind of living with the reality of FA and the emotional toll of it all saps your energy and eats away at your time. Fortunately, though, God will be the judge of everything, and I'm grateful for that, because he is all-seeing, all-knowing and understands each of us and what drives us in this sometimes-difficult life. Most importantly I feel at peace with him.

Major surgery

12

Once we left the hospital after speaking to the scoliosis surgeon I decided to do some research. I was mulling over the questions about blood, and they continued to hang over me for many months. In the meantime I decided to find out what I could about scoliosis.

We had attended the hospital that served our area for spinal surgery. It was based just over an hour away in Birmingham. The surgeon that we saw was a lovely man who knew his operating team well. He knew that his anaesthetist would not entertain the idea of bloodless surgery in Krystie's case. They considered that she was a high-risk operating subject. The risks were:

- They needed to open Krystie's back from top to bottom.
- They intended to fuse each vertebrae to the next one.
- Her heart was enlarged on its left side causing an irregular heart rhythm; the length of the operation (approximately seven hours) would put pressure on her heart.
- People with FA have weaker muscle tone, and when their muscles are cut they have the propensity to actually pump blood out, unlike our muscles which usually contract and thereby help to stem the flow of blood a little.
- FA is an illness that produces different effects in every person who has it, therefore operating on an FA patient is charting unknown territory, so to speak.

I could see their point. I began my research. I searched the Internet and found out all about the operation. Next I contacted several specialist hospitals in America and talked to them about our situation. The doctors were in all cases really helpful. When I left messages for people they returned my calls. No one was judgemental and they were all helpful. Once I was sure in my mind about the medical facts, I started to search the Internet for information about UK hospitals and doctors. On the website for spinal studies I came across a surgeon based in Nottingham. I contacted his secretary, got their email details, and then emailed him with my experience to date. I received a prompt reply and made an appointment to visit him. I paid privately for the initial consultation and took Krystie up to see him. A few weeks before our appointment I telephoned our Birmingham hospital and requested that they forward all of Krystie's X-rays to Nottingham so that the surgeon could look at them in advance.

This particular surgeon had been operating on spines for over twenty years and was very experienced. He had also operated on Jehovah's Witnesses without using blood, and was happy to do it again. He didn't share the same view as the Birmingham surgeon. Whilst he agreed that the operation was risky, he explained that he would use all the blood-saving techniques that he could, and would also use a cell-saver machine. His other comments were that if at any time he felt Krystie was at risk he would simply stop the operation and stitch her back up. He agreed that operations carry many risks, severe blood loss being one of them. Krystie still had the heart risk and the paralysis risk. In spite of those things Krystie and I both left his consulting room that afternoon feeling happy with his views. I told him that I would approach Birmingham and ask them to transfer the funding for Krystie's operation so that we could have the surgery up at Nottingham. The surgeon agreed to take her on.

Anthony was getting ready to go travelling around Australia and South East Asia. He was obviously excited, but just a few days before he left we were in the garden. It was a beautiful hot day; I looked at him sitting thoughtfully by the pond and went to ask him what he was thinking about. To my surprise he was actually quite emotional. 'What's the matter?' I asked. He looked at me and said, 'It's not fair mom, look at me about to go off on a fantastic trip while Krystie gets ready for an operation. Will she ever be able to do the things that me and Nik have done, will she?' Of course I felt choked, but I calmly said that he needed to just live his life and not worry about Krystie. I told him that she didn't expect him to worry about her and, furthermore, none of us knew what Krystie would eventually do, but I had a feeling that she would surprise the lot of us. I also said that if she wanted to go travelling then she could, she would just achieve it in a slightly different way. I told him to go and enjoy his trip and then come back and tell us all what he'd experienced because we would all enjoy hearing about his exploits. It was a reminder that all of us have our days when the sadness overwhelms you; I just wished that my children didn't have to experience them.

I wrote to the Birmingham hospital and explained how I felt. I thanked them for their care, but explained that I needed Krystie to have her operation performed by a team that started it in the belief that it was going to be OK. In my mind, if a team started the operation believing that she would probably die on the operating table, then it wasn't the place that I needed them to be. I did, however, thank them for their honesty, and understood that this was about the differences in people, experience and the whole team. The Birmingham team anaesthetist wrote to Krystie and me and asked us to go in and talk to him, which we did. He was a lovely, humble man. He asked Krystie what her views were, and she eloquently explained how she felt, what she believed, and why. What she said and how she explained it was very moving even to me. He thanked her, and explained that he had been practising for several years, but that in terms of experience he didn't feel confident that he could manage her surgery without blood. He said that to do so required a level of skill that he didn't have yet. I explained that I had been up to Nottingham and that they had said that they were willing to carry out the operation without blood. He said that if they were confident then we should go to Nottingham, and he would write to them and ask if he could go and watch some operations without using blood because it was a skill that he would like to develop. That is why I considered him to be humble – he didn't have to spend time talking to us did he? He could have just said that he wasn't willing to carry out the operation but he didn't. He was obviously a man who genuinely cared. So I never felt that Birmingham was a lesser team. I have always understood that our request pushes medicine to its limits, their honesty was because they wanted the best outcome for Krystie, and they were willing to accept that on this occasion with this set of circumstances Nottingham was the best option. He said that he would let the relevant hospital people know that he was backing our decision to transfer Krystie's case.

All we had to do was sit back and wait for the surgery date to be scheduled. It was September 2004 and we were told that the waiting list was between eight and ten months. Krystie returned to school to start yet another year; the difference was that she was starting her GCSE courses, so it was a key year. I wasn't sure how she would cope with all of this worry hanging over her but she seemed to.

Krystie and I had stayed in touch with Min Clough over the intervening years; she really is a lovely lady, and she got on very well with Krystie. Sometime during that autumn I met up with Min in London when I was working on a project. It was lovely to see her and, as always, I gave her an update on Krystie. She was shocked to learn about the impending operation. Min had always said that she would like to make a follow-up programme about Krystie, and she said that she thought this whole experience might make an interesting one. My initial reaction was 'no'. I felt that the operation was risky and that the outcome was uncertain and so did not like the idea of it being filmed. I hadn't really considered Krystie's view. When I got home that evening and chatted about the day with her, I told her about my meeting with Min. I told her that she had said that she thought the situation we were living through at this time might make an interesting programme. However, I said that I thought it was too risky to film us, because we could not guarantee the outcome. 'Excuse me mother, but I would definitely like to make the programme; people should know what we have to live through!' I looked at her, 'Yes I can see that, but Krystie what if the operation goes wrong?' Krystie rolled her eyes at me, 'So what? This is my life, that is what could happen, and I have to live with that; like I say, other people should know what goes on in our lives.' She was adamant that she wanted to do it. I contacted Min to let her know that I had been overruled and that Krystie did in fact want to make the programme. Min was pleased, and said that we should really think about it. She also needed to make sure that the programme could be signed off. We agreed to talk again in a few weeks' time, which we did, when we agreed to make the programme

Early in 2005 Krystie discovered McFly. She drove the entire family completely nuts with her McFly obsession. I couldn't believe it; one minute she had been mad about Julie Andrews, and now it was McFly! Not much difference between the two!? She played their music constantly at full blast. I spent most of my time asking her to turn the music down. It was annoying, but also nice to see her in good spirits. She was to all intents and purposes a normal teenage girl and yet she was living under this enormous pressure. She didn't really seem to mind. Personally I felt like a pressure cooker about to explode. I found that even though I appeared normal, my breath felt quite short and I always felt on ten-terhooks. Everything we did was tinged with sadness. I found myself wondering if those things we did together would be the last. I felt like her days were numbered, and it was killing me.

Nicholas and Stephanie announced that they were expecting their first baby. Krystie was really pleased, she couldn't wait to meet her new nephew, who was due in June. Odd things cross your mind. I found myself thinking about the old wives' tale, which says that a birth follows a death. I couldn't believe myself.

In the springtime, I contacted the hospital to find out if they had scheduled a date for Krystie's surgery and I was told that they were just about to write to us to give us a date for May. I explained that I didn't really want the operation to happen in May because I had booked three weeks off work in July and we were all due to be going out to Portugal. If the operation could be scheduled for July, then my little ones could go ahead with the holiday and travel with my sister's family and I could spend the time I needed to up in Nottingham with Krystie. The lady said that she usually got asked to cancel dates so that people could travel, not so that people could cancel their holidays! She understood my reasoning and promised to do her best. About two weeks later I got a date within a few days of my original request, 18 July. Perfect.

One evening I was reading through the local newspaper when I noticed that McFly were due to visit our town and play at the Civic Hall. I got us some tickets and told Krystie that she would be going to see them. She was ecstatic. I secretly emailed the Civic Hall and told them all about Krystie and asked them if they could arrange for her to meet McFly. I didn't hear anything for a few days, but then I got a message to say that the promoters were considering the request and would let us know nearer the date. I could hardly believe it, and somehow managed to keep it to myself. About a week before the concert, Krystie came home from school and told me that her support assistant, who helped when and if she needed it at school, had written to the Civic Hall to ask them if they could arrange for her to meet McFly. I couldn't believe it. So the Civic Hall had had two requests, one from me, and one from her teacher! The day of the concert finally arrived. I spoke with the public relations office who told me that McFly's management were still considering my request, and they would let me know later on in the afternoon. He also said that they had turned down every other request except ours; even the local newspaper had been refused, so it looked very promising. Krystie also had her annual heart check-up on that day. I had rearranged the appointment to ensure that we would be out of Birmingham and on our way home by 3 p.m. It was good news. We were told that her heart function was the same as the previous year, which was good. I asked the heart team to copy the results to Nottingham for me so that they would have them on record for the impending operation.

Krystie and I set off on our journey home. She was like a bottle of pop, so excited she couldn't wait for the evening to arrive. I had told her that I was trying to arrange for her to meet the lads, but she knew that we were still waiting for a definite answer. As we were driving along, my car telephone rang; I took the call. It was the Civic Hall, calling to say that McFly would love to meet Krystie. They asked us to meet their security staff at a side entrance thirty minutes before the show started. I ended the call and we both started screaming! I don't know why I was, but I just felt so happy for her. We called Min to share the good news; Krystie was screaming down the phone mike. Min got really excited too. She said she wished she could join us, because we had passed the 'excitement' bug to her. She then asked me if there was any way that I could record Krystie, because she would like to capture the mood she was in that day. I said that of course I would. We got home and then got changed to go out. Krystie was glowing. Mitch took us up to town. We waited at the side door as requested, and the security men came to meet us. They took us up to the seats and told us that they would come back for us when McFly were ready to meet Krystie. About ten minutes later they came and took us into a side room. Krystie sat in her wheelchair, and one of the management team spoke to us, then suddenly a curtain moved and McFly were filing into the room smiling. They all greeted Krystie with a kiss on the cheek and spoke to her. For the only time in her life I witnessed Krystie speechless, she couldn't talk. She kept trying to talk but kept forgetting her words, she was clearly star-struck. After a few minutes she regained her composure and managed to utter a few phrases. To this day she is sure that the guys must think she was completely mad! She wishes she could have spoken to them properly! I asked them if they would pose for photos, which they did, so we captured the moment for posterity. They gave her a plectrum and a pair of drumsticks, which really surprised her. We rejoined the auditorium and Krystie was practically mobbed by excited teenagers asking her if 'she had just met them!' One girl asked her if she had kissed them and practically swooned when Krystie said 'yes'. It was so funny. The concert began and Krystie watched it from her own cloud nine. I thought that they were lovely to agree to meet Krystie. They didn't do it for the publicity, simply because they wanted to meet her. I became a fan of theirs from that day!

It was May now, so well and truly spring. July was approaching more quickly than we had anticipated. My grandson Tyler arrived on 4 June. He was beautiful and Krystie loved him. He was a light in the dark tunnel that we were all in at that time.

The kids were fine; Mitch and I were not. I was a bag of nerves, and Mitch was dreading the prospect of hospitals. He was irritated by everything and I knew that he just wanted to get away from it all. I was annoyed because I felt that no one had asked for this but we just had to get through it. We were completely out of sync with each other and we knew it. We just didn't know what to do about it. So we did nothing. At the back of my mind, I knew what the problem was, and I felt that everything would get back to normal after the operation. Anybody would have found the situation stressful I'm sure.

The BBC crew came to see us, and capture some film. In one way it was good for Krystie to have the distraction, and the ability to talk to an outsider is as good as a counselling session I think. Min talks to Krystie a lot, and is objective. She also treats Krystie with respect. She is very good for her.

In mid-June we were invited to the hospital so that Krystie could have some pre-operative assessments. We agreed that the BBC could film us. They contacted the hospital and also obtained permission from them. On the actual day our surgeon was busy and came to meet us in between clinic and surgery. We had not seen him for several months but due to lack of time the only chance that we had to speak to him was in front of the camera. He surprised us by saying that he had checked Krystie's X-rays again, and had decided he could approach the operation in a different way. It seemed that the curve was like an S-shape; but the surgical team believed that the main curve was at the base of Krystie's spine and this curve was throwing the top of the spine out in a compensatory movement. Therefore if they could fuse the base of the spine, the top half would be stable. Taking this approach meant that they could perform the operation from the front of Krystie's body rather than the back (anterior). Making the incision from the front was much much safer because they would not have to cut through muscle and therefore the blood loss would be reduced. It also meant that she didn't have to have her back cut open from top to bottom, or the entire length of her spine fused. It seemed like a much better option to me. It was as if someone had taken a magic wand and removed nearly twelve months of worry. He repeated that he did not think for one minute that blood would be an issue in this surgery. He felt that it would be straightforward. Krystie and I didn't quite know what to make of it all, but were really pleased.

We also had to meet the consultant anaesthetist. He came to see us and introduced himself. Again on camera he asked us about the operation. It became clear that he had a different opinion to the surgeon and was more worried about the prospect of not using blood, especially because of Krystie's age. He was also concerned about the fact that the operation was going to be filmed. During the interview I answered a question by telling him I was divorced from Krystie's father; I could tell by his reaction that he was a bit concerned by that. He asked me about custody and I explained that I had care and control of the children. He asked Krystie if she was worried about the surgery and she said, 'Look I am one person who has FA, and I have to manage that, but I am only "one" person. The illness affects only me. But if you look around the world, there are things happening that affect so many people and that's what I worry about – NOT ME.' I was so touched; I had a lump in my throat. She was amazing. The filming stopped, he was friendly and said we shouldn't worry and then left. Krystie and I were still on a high, and so we went along to our next appointment of the day with a spring in our step (and wheels).

The next appointment was with a person who wired Krystie up to a machine with electrodes. The electrodes picked up signals down her main nerve pathways and gave readings that could then be used to track her condition during surgery. The purpose of the readings was to protect her spinal cord. It was my understanding that the surgeon would monitor the readings during the operation to ensure that Krystie's cord was not damaged. They wired her up using this awful glue to stick the electrodes onto her scalp. I wondered how we would ever get the gunk out of her hair. Krystie, who is extremely ticklish, wriggled and screamed all over the place, as they tried to stick the electrodes to her arms and legs. Once Krystie starts giggling, she cannot stop and ends up shrieking with laughter. She ended up getting told off and finally tried really hard to suppress her giggles and keep still so that they could finish the job. Min and I were trying hard not to laugh too, but it was a comical scene. When she was ready they switched on the machine and it started to do its job. Unfortunately they could not get the readings that they needed; I wasn't surprised because I knew that her nerve pathways had broken down, which is why she can't walk, but I had hoped they might get something. This meant that they would do the operation 'in the dark' as it were, with nothing to monitor her spinal cord at all. As far as I was concerned this was the biggest risk that we had to worry about, not the blood.

The next day, the anaesthetist called me and what he had to say threw me in to a bit of a panic. Basically he said that because Krystie was only 15 and we were intending to have the operation filmed he was feeling quite concerned. He felt that if anything went wrong he was leaving himself wide open to litigation. He was also concerned because I was divorced from Krystie's father. He said that he needed proof that I did have 'care and control' of the children before he would agree to operating without blood. I talked to him about the changes to the planned operation and how the surgeon had said that he was not worried at all. He replied that it was his job to keep Krystie alive; and that with her FA, enlarged heart, seven hours of surgery and her being a minor he was not taking it lightly. I promised him that I would contact my solicitor to get a copy of my divorce papers.

I called the solicitors' office and asked to speak to the secretary. I explained the situation and requested a copy of my papers. She took my details and said she would call me back. A couple of hours later she called to say that they could not find my paperwork, and that in view of the dates it was likely they had been destroyed. I could not believe this was happening. Not now, just two weeks before the surgery. She explained there were some boxes of papers in a locked room that were due to be destroyed and the key holder would be back in the office the next day when they could check to see if my papers were amongst them. She added that she thought it was unlikely. I just put the phone down and told myself to stay calm because all I could do was wait. The next day she phoned to let me know that they had found my papers in those boxes after all. I breathed a sigh of relief that I had been saved by the skin of my teeth. However, the next part of her sentence took my breath away. She explained that it seemed that the paragraphs concerning my children had not been drawn up as I expected, and therefore I did not have the sole right to make medical decisions about them. I was flabbergasted, because I had brought them up under the misapprehension that I did have custody of them. The past was irrelevant now, but under these circumstances it was vital and important. I asked her to fax through a letter from the solicitor explaining the divorce and stating what my rights were. Once I received it, I faxed it over to the hospital. As I expected, the anaesthetist called me to say that he could not agree to me signing the papers to request bloodless surgery because he felt that if anything went wrong Krystie's father could sue him. He said that he would like to speak to my ex-husband and obtain his permission to my request.

I explained that I did not want him to contact my ex because I did not believe that he had the right to have any say whatsoever in her medical treatment. This is because he had never ever attended one hospital or doctor's appointment, not one. Once, quite soon after Krystie had been diagnosed, I had been really poorly, so I had asked him to take her to one of her London appointments, but he wouldn't, so my mother had to take her instead. As I spoke, he had not been in contact with Krystie for over three months, not even a phone call. It stuck in my throat to think that he could offer any sort of opinion to do with the care of Krystie. I said that I needed to think, and that I would call back the next day. I put a call in to the surgeon to explain what had happened. He said that he could not understand why everything was getting so complicated. He said that he was virtually 100 per cent convinced that blood would not be an issue in this surgery, and he assured me that he had no intention of using it. I trusted him, and I believed him.

The legal department of the hospital spoke with me later that day. It seemed that legally they had to contact Krystie's father if I insisted that the surgery go ahead without blood. If they spoke to him about the situation and he refused to agree with me, then they would have to go to court to get a judge to rule. It was likely that in the case of a minor, even an eloquent assertive minor, he would rule in her father's favour. Furthermore, if her father ever raised the question of FA perhaps affecting Krystie's ability to make mature decisions I would stand virtually no chance of the judge ruling on my side. Most important of all, at this late stage such an argument would delay her operation for a few months.

Krystie was very happy that she was having the operation in the summer holidays because it meant that she could return to school in September and begin her examination studies. I knew that if she thought for one minute that her operation was going to be delayed she would be devastated. If I could have trusted her father to agree with us, then I might have asked him; but I didn't. A few years earlier he had stated in no uncertain terms that if she ever needed blood he would let her have it. I wished that Krystie was 16 but she wasn't, she was 15; just those few months could have made quite a difference. It seemed that had she been 16 that they would have been willing to accept the decision in her own right.

The legal person suggested that perhaps we approach the problem in a different way. She explained that the surgeon was sure he would not use blood; his opinion was that catastrophic blood loss was highly unlikely and he did not think for one minute that we would need blood. The anaesthetist agreed that it was unlikely, but preferred to cover himself in case of litigation especially since Krystie was a minor, and her father was divorced from me. He had said that he was willing to go ahead with the surgery if I allowed them to write a statement to the affect that both Krystie and I requested strongly that the surgery be performed without using whole blood. We would accept blood substitutes and permitted components, agree to the use of a cell saver and understand that all medical personnel would do their utmost to work within these boundaries. However, if they considered that Krystie's life was in danger they would have to use blood. Basically they were asking for a get-out clause.

I cleared my mind, and tried to take all of the emotion out of everything. The facts were that Krystie's operation had been changed; she was now due to undergo anterior scoliosis surgery, which meant that blood loss would be minimal. The surgeon who had over twenty years experience in this field was assuring me that in his opinion it was highly unlikely blood would even be an issue. Now the anaesthetist was saying that it was unlikely that she would lose a lot of blood, but in this litigious climate he wanted to be sure that he could not be sued in the future. My divorce papers had not been drawn up correctly and therefore I wasn't in a legal position to make demands. In the cold light of day, I realised that I could fight on principle but that would mean postponing the operation and going to court. At the end of it all I would be in exactly the same situation that I was in right now. I thought long and hard, I prayed long and hard. I spoke to the surgeon again, and he assured me that blood would not be an issue. I trusted him. From the moment I met him I had felt comfortable with him. Actually a throwaway comment by the matron on his ward sealed my final decision. I was chatting generally with her about the surgery, and I said that there had been a bit of a disagreement over the blood. She looked at me and said, 'We avoid using blood with children as much as possible anyway.' That was it, I agreed to sign the papers as they recommended. I did it because I believed that it wouldn't be a problem.

That weekend, we had a family get together. We had a meal in the garden, and I had a photographer come over to take some pictures. I had this overwhelming need to have some photos of me with both of my girls, and then some photos of all the children together. We had a really beautiful day. The BBC came along to film part of it too. It was so nice to have that calm afternoon together. Her operation was just days away, so we savoured every moment.

The next weekend arrived far too quickly. Krystie and I drove up to the hospital on the Sunday ready for her to 'check in' for 'D' day, which was to be the Monday. It took us about an hour and a half to get there. We listened to McFly and talked about the operation. Eventually we arrived on the ward. As we walked in the nurse looked at us and said 'Didn't you get a call?' I looked at her questioningly. She said, 'I think that they have cancelled your operation.' Krystie half spoke, half cried, 'No, they can't have, not after all this, no please no.' She was really upset and tears were rolling down her cheeks. The nurse said that she would go and find out what was going on. I told her that I had telephoned at 4.30 p.m. on Friday to check that it was still scheduled and had been told yes. We sat in the waiting room for what seemed like forever. Krystie was destroyed. I think that she had geared herself up for it and now the emotion was coming out. Eventually the nurse came back. It was all right, they would do it after all; she was apologetic and pleased for us. To this day, I am still not sure about what happened. I was that relieved that I didn't have the strength to demand an explanation. We went to our room and got settled in. The anaesthetist came to bring the paperwork for us to sign. The statement had been drafted so that he was happy with it. We both signed the forms. He thanked us and, as he left, he said that he was 99 per cent sure that actually there was not going to be a problem, but he just felt he had to protect himself. Next the surgeon's registrar came.

We signed their paperwork too and I noticed that the wording was slightly different but in the same vein as the first lot of forms. Again he assured me that the surgeon had no intention of using blood.

I had a camp bed in Krystie's room; we decided to get an early night because we were going down to theatre at 6.45 the next morning. I telephoned Mitch to let him know, because he was joining me in the morning and bringing my mom. I also spoke to my boys and asked them to tell their dad so that he could get to the hospital in time. He hadn't spoken to Krystie for over three months, but I knew that he would want to see her before she went under. Surprisingly we both slept well, and before we knew it the nurses were waking us to get ready to be taken down. Krystie showered and changed into a gown.

The BBC arrived. They were going to be filming the whole operation. I walked alongside her bed as they wheeled her down. It's a strange feeling; everyone is trying to be upbeat when really all you feel is anxiety. However, we arrived at theatre and waited to be told to enter the ante-room. We all put sterile gowns on. Krystie was amazing; she was cracking jokes and was very upbeat. Her attitude lifted everyone's spirits. Then we got the nod to enter the ante-room. The anaesthetist was sitting with his gown and mask on. He prepared her and then administered the 'knockout' drugs. He looked at me, 'Give her a kiss, mom', which I did, and then he said 'Count backwards from 10, Krystie' – 10, 9, 8, 7, 6 . . . she was gone. It was that quick. The nurse took my arm, 'Come on mom, let's go and wait upstairs.' As we walked back to the ward, the nurse looked at me and said, 'I have never known anyone so calm and so chirpy whilst waiting for major surgery, she is amazing.' I could see that she was really touched.

I didn't feel anything really. It was surreal, so calm. I couldn't make sense of it. One minute walking down, then Krystie laughing, then gone. I went back upstairs, and by now my mother and Mitch had arrived. They were disappointed that they had missed her, but traffic had been bad, and then Krystie had actually been taken down slightly earlier than we had anticipated. I told them not to worry, because they had both seen her the day before, and waved her off from home. We all went for a cup of tea. You wonder what you can do for seven hours. Your child's life in someone else's hands. We talked, we drank tea. I looked at the photos that had been taken just over a week ago. It was all so false, like it wasn't happening to you. We went to sit in her room and wait. At about eleven o'clock her dad arrived with Anthony. He was disappointed that he had missed her. I didn't have one word to say about that, because I had sent a message about the time.

We all sat together. The clock ticked away. Actually in some ways, it went quite quickly, and it wasn't as bad as I had expected it to be. Then it got to six hours, and I started to feel odd. The last hour seemed to go really slowly, and then it was finally gone. So now we were going into eight hours, and I started to feel panic. Everyone had talked about a seven-hour operation not eight, so what was happening. Was she OK? I went to talk to one of the crew on camera, and then suddenly saw Anthony and the surgeon walking towards me. I didn't know what to think, searching his face for a clue, and then he smiled, 'She's fine Mrs Maddox, it went well, no problems and we didn't use blood, in fact she hardly lost any blood at all.' I didn't know whether to laugh or cry but I felt good.

I just wanted to see her; I wanted to hug her and look at her, but we had to wait. The film crew came up. They told me that the operation had been marvellous. They told me that at one point the operating team had even brought Krystie out of the anaesthetic so that they could ask her to wiggle her toes. They wanted to check her spinal cord; once she had wiggled them they knew that her cord was fine and put her back to sleep. Amazing. But we still couldn't see her. Everyone was smiling and laughing, the pressure lifted. My brave girl. The call came through. We could make our way over to the high-dependency unit in intensive care. We started on the walk over to see her. When we arrived, it all seemed a little bit chaotic. Once they let us on to the ward they asked us to sit in a side room, explaining that they had a medical emergency with another patient to deal with and so asked us to bear with them whilst they sorted it out. We sat patiently and waited some more. It was awful. Then they came and said that we could go and see her two at a time. I went to see her with Mitch. She was wired up to this machine, and everything was bleeping. I stroked her gently and called her name. She half-opened her eyes, and muttered, 'I made it.' It was so good to see her, and know that she was OK. We went to swap over with Anthony and his dad and as we left the ward I noticed a medical emergency: she was a small blonde girl, lying on a bed surrounded by at least five nurses. She looked bruised and blotchy, and I knew immediately that she had meningitis. It was a sorry sight. She looked very young, only about 3 or 4.

Krystie

The operation was hard on me. The last thing I thought before I was put under was about my nephew, Tyler. I thought, okay, you gotta get through this Krystie, you've got a nephew now, and if you don't make it back he won't even remember you! So I woke up and though I was exhausted and in a horrendous amount of pain, I felt happy and lucky.

Again filming was fun, and it was great seeing Min again, I do love making documentaries.

Eventually my family visitors left, and I went back to Krystie. I sat with her. When she woke a little I asked her if she could remember who had visited her just a few hours previously, when she first arrived back from surgery. As I went through the names she nodded to each one, then she moved her oxygen mask, and asked, 'Was everyone all right with seeing me in here (intensive care)? They weren't too worried by all of this were they?' I could not believe that in her delicate half-awake state she was still more concerned with others than herself. Next she said, 'When I woke up after the operation, I was so glad that I was still alive!' I knew it, she had been really worried, but she had put on a brave face, bless her.

I sat with her for the next couple of hours. It was an amazing ward. Every patient had their own dedicated nurse who stood by them monitoring them constantly. Krystie was not filling her lungs with air properly, and so the machine was bleeping every few minutes. I was worried at first, but you get used to it. I kept talking to Krystie, coaxing her to take deep breaths. I stood right next to her, and watched the machine like a hawk. Every time her oxygen dropped I talked to her and encouraged her to breathe deeply. She was moaning with pain, it really hurt her to breathe. It was not surprising really because they had removed a rib (which they crushed and mixed with a glue-like substance to pack her spine) and they had also deflated her lung so that they could actually get to her spine in order to operate. They had removed five discs at the bottom. It was incredible to think what she had been through. She had a chest drain, which is a tube about the diameter of a 20p piece, inserted through her side and it really hurt her. It was hard to watch her, and hear her cry out in agony. You just wanted to take the pain away, but her nurse said that it was really important that she breathed properly and really filled her lungs. Eventually she fell into a sleep, and so I left her to go and get some sleep myself. The next morning I sat with her again. The little blonde girl was still critical; she had six people monitoring her constantly she was so poorly. After a few hours, they told me that Krystie was stable enough to go back to the ward. They explained that she would be in a high-dependency bed, and so be monitored closely. I felt nervous about leaving intensive care, they were so fantastic in there, but I knew that she was stable and so well enough to transfer.

Over the course of the next few days Krystie grew stronger and stronger. She was quiet and she slept a lot but she looked fairly well. I just sat with her and made sure she ate something and drank a little. The pain did get her down, but on the whole she did well. She was moved out of the high-dependency bay and back into her own room. She was pleased about that. She had been in hospital about a week now. She had asked Min not to come and film her just after the operation because she didn't want to be on camera looking really poorly; Min respected her wishes.

I decided to pop home. I wanted to get Krystie's room sorted out ready for her return. The decorator had been in and repainted her room, Mitch had bought her a new TV and had it mounted on a stand, which he fitted to the wall. He had also bought a Freeview box. I went out and bought her a new duvet, cushions and accessories. Her room looked beautiful, ready for her to come home. I spent one night at home working with Mitch to get everything sorted out, and then I went back to the hospital.

Krystie stayed in hospital for nearly three weeks. She was very weak at first, and scared to try and do things, probably because she did feel weak. She knows that her legs are weak, and so she was reluctant to try and take her weight on them in case they gave way. In her head, I think she thought her back would break if she fell. This meant that I was taking a lot of her weight when she needed to transfer on to a bed pan, or use the shower. I was rolling her over to get her dressed and quite often I was alone. Hospitals are very busy, and when parents are about I think that you can get left to get on with things. I ended up straining my back. I was really in agony. So I drove home to have another night there, in order to rest. It was the best thing that I could have done. I felt really guilty about leaving Krystie but I needed to get some rest. She hates being dependant on others. She didn't mind me helping her, but she knew that if she didn't try hard she would be reliant on everyone else to do things for her. For example rather than lift her or take her weight the nurses used a hoist to lift her, and she hated it. So when I wasn't there she pushed herself with gritty determination to roll over, and then stand with support. Once she made her mind up to do it, there was no stopping her. 'Mom, I just want to get home,' she said when I got back. 'I really do want to go home.'

One day I left the ward to go and fetch a coffee, and bumped into the nurse from the intensive care unit. She asked me how Krystie was doing and I told her very well. I also asked her about the little blonde girl. She looked at me and said, 'Oh, she died.' I felt terrible. To think that she was such a little girl who would have been so perfect just a few days ago, and yet she was dead. I remember thinking about my conversations with Krystie and I thought to myself that yes, life really does take unexpected twists. I felt terrible for her parents, I really did.

I was reminded of this again later that day when I bumped into one of the other moms whose daughter had had similar surgery to Krystie. Her spinal cord had been injured, and so it was uncertain as to whether or not she was going to be able to walk again. She was only 10 or 11. She didn't have any kind of genetic illness, just scoliosis. A different surgeon had carried out her surgery and unfortunately something had gone wrong. Despite the fact that the spinal cord monitor worked perfectly on her, something had gone wrong. What can I say? You can never tell, can you. The hospital discharged us, and we made the journey home. We took it really steady because every bump in the road meant pain for Krystie. She didn't know whether to laugh or cry. In fact we both ended up laughing because it was like a comedy sketch. I crawled along the roads while Krystie winced in the back! The BBC were waiting to film the homecoming. It was very peaceful. Harrison and McKenna were out in Portugal with my sister and her family and Anthony was at work. So it was just Mitch and I (and the cameras). I preferred it that way. I just wanted to get her settled and comfortable. She loved her room and TV and was very, very happy to be home.

Krystie was in a lot of pain initially and slept for very long periods. The nerves at the top of her legs seemed to play up, and she literally sobbed with the pain some days. But as usual she was brave. She wanted to do everything for herself, and hated me fussing. By the middle of August the children came back, and the house was full of hustle and bustle again. After living under so much stress for so long it was like a breath of fresh air to feel normal again. The physiotherapists visited us and worked with Krystie to get her stronger. She found the exercises hard but she did her best. She was very tired and continued to sleep for long periods of time. She was taking lots of painkillers and was in considerable pain, but she didn't really moan. She decided that she didn't like taking all the painkillers, and so started her own reduction programme. I couldn't believe it, but she wanted to stop taking them. I thought that she was incredibly brave.

I had expected her to stay at home for a few weeks, but she was sure that she wanted to return to school at the start of the new term. I contacted the school, and although they were shocked they were pleased too. I spoke with Jane Sellar who went to talk to the school to advise them on the best way to support Krystie. I had my reservations, but have learned with Krystie that it's best to let her make her own decisions. If she makes a mistake, she realises, and isn't too proud to admit it. So she did return to school in the first week of term. She actually joined her friends two days into the new term, as the school had requested that she allow them two days to make sure that all the pupils knew that they were not to touch her wheelchair.

She arrived home after her first day, jubilant that she had made it. Her strength amazed me and humbled me all at the same time. At the end of the second week, I knew that Krystie was shattered, and I spoke to the school, who felt the same. Krystie was collapsing into bed when she got back from school and sleeping until the next morning. We all spoke to her about the operation, and her remarkable efforts, but we also told her that she really needed time to heal. So we eventually agreed to a reduced week for Krystie. She went to school for one whole day, three half days and took Fridays off. Krystie was really worried about her exams, due in summer 2006, but knew that she was incredibly tired. Once again she didn't really have a choice. After just one week of the new arrangements, you could see the colour come back to her cheeks. Following the surgery she lost about two stones in weight, which was a lot because she wasn't big before the operation. But somehow, she started to look stronger.

Jane, the physio, and Gail, from wheelchair services, came out to see us. They wanted to make some changes to her electric chair following the surgery. Krystie got really upset and actually shouted at everybody. 'Just leave me alone, why can't you? Do you know what it's like when you use an electric chair? People don't see you. Now you are asking me to use it with changes that I know will make people stare at me. I don't want too. I'm sick of people seeing my chair; I just want them to see me!! I like the chair that mom and dad bought me.' She was very emotional and crying. We were all shocked at her outburst; she can be outspoken but she doesn't usually shout at people. However, the medics all put their heads together to see what they could do with Krystie's chair to make it more acceptable to her. They understood what she meant but were trying to balance the support of her back post-surgery and her weak muscles with a practical chair. They agreed to go away and come up with a solution.

We arranged a special treat for Krystie. McFly were in concert at Nottingham, so I arranged to have a limousine pick her up along with three friends. We took them to the concert in style. They loved every minute of it. Krystie felt like a celebrity. It was wonderful to watch her with her friends, it really was. Before we knew it we were once again approaching the end of another year. Krystie grew stronger and stronger, and looked really well again. The wheelchair was adapted and modified to be much more acceptable to Krystie. She is much happier with it now.

Min (from the BBC) managed to get Krystie tickets to sit in the audience to watch an audience with Dame Julie Andrews. Can you believe it! She was ecstatic, yet another hero that she got to see. She really enjoyed it. She continues to blast out McFly and all the other music that she likes, and like any other teenager drives me to distraction.

At the beginning of 2006, Krystie increased her school week so that she was attending two full days and three half days. She felt much better about that, and though she still worries about her exams, feels that she should get the results that she wants.

When I think about everything that's happened, I can't quite believe it. As for the future – who knows? I remember myself as a child full of so much happiness that at times I was ready to burst. I faced my future with so much optimism. But, then what would any of us do if we knew our futures?

Anthony's memories 13

The family was growing. Harrison had been born during the previous year, a baby in the house again after so many years. We had just settled into our own first house. We had finally started to feel like a family, everyone settled in their lives . . . then the bombshell was dropped!

Krystie had been taken to a swimming lesson by my mom. They both returned and my mom looked distressed. The swimming instructor had challenged my mom about Krystie's illness – the illness we didn't even know existed – and had brashly asked her why she hadn't made her aware of it. My mom, confused by this question, replied that there was no illness. The instructor dismissed this possibility as she felt that there was definitely something wrong with Krystie and we had to find out what.

In a way we had known for a few years! Krystie was tiny. She walked awkwardly, couldn't run properly, and shook when carrying something.

My mom had taken her for testing for multiple conditions, but they always came back negative. Since the doctors could not find anything wrong my mom was convinced that it was all in her own head. Nicholas and I never discussed there being anything wrong with Krystie. Personally I knew there was something not quite right, her body was not in 'sync', it wasn't operating or developing correctly.

I used to put these thoughts and worries to the back of my mind clinging to the hope that I was mistaken, and that in fact Krystie was fine.

After the swimming pool incident, when it became clear that a detailed investigation into Krystie was going to take place, I didn't want it to. My opinion was that in this matter ignorance was bliss. I didn't want to know what was wrong with Krystie because I knew it was going to shake all our lives to the core. It's one thing suspecting that your little sister has an illness, an entirely different thing knowing it and having to deal with it. To have to see her life crushed like I suspected was going to be too hard to handle. At the age of 14 I had no idea how I would ever deal with it . . .

So she had it. Friedreich's Ataxia. A completely incurable, untreatable, genetic illness. This was the worst of the scenarios that we had considered. Option one was a brain tumour, meaning a big operation, a difficult year, but at the end of the day likely a cured Krystie who could look forward to leading a normal life in the future. Option two was the genetic illness, unbeatable, uncom-promising, a hopeless case! To add insult to injury, it was caused by faulty genes in my parents, meaning Krystie had been doomed from day one!

I opened the door to Krystie when she returned with my mom from the visit to the hospital on the day that they more or less confirmed that she did have the disease. She looked up at me, smiled, and said, 'Well Ant, looks like I've got it, Friedreich's Ataxia.' I didn't know what to say. I simply returned to my cereal which I had been interrupted from eating. I've never been 'a crier' at emotionally hard times. When I was told by my mom that her and my dad were to divorce, I didn't cry, I just said 'okay' and after a chat with my mom, went to bed. This was a similar moment, a moment when I should have broken down with sadness but instead I just ate my cereal and stared into space.

Krystie followed me into the kitchen and challenged me, 'Well don't you care, Ant?' I replied, 'Of course I do'. But I could muster no more words to say to her. I felt numb; I felt numbness for a long time.

As we already knew what Friedreich's Ataxia entailed, we knew that Krystie's illness was for the long term. It wasn't something that could be fixed, and it wasn't something that acted quickly and violently. We were going to have to slowly watch Krystie get worse and worse. It was for this reason that I felt I couldn't break down.

We had to get on with it; it was as simple as that. Though I was disgusted and upset for Krystie, I felt that I had to treat her normally to ensure that she continued to grow in her life, to develop as a person, and enjoy her life to the greatest extent possible.

I can gladly say that, to date, she has done just that. She has been in mainstream school throughout, mixing with able-bodied children every day. She has starred in two television programmes, and has recently auditioned for a part in a BBC television drama series, which I pray that she gets.

I am very proud of how my family has moved forward from that day when we found out about Krystie's illness. None of us stood and moped about what we had found out. We attacked the future fearlessly. A new home was bought, with a swimming pool to help Krystie keep her mobility. There was a new addition to the family in McKenna, and Nicholas met the girl who was to become his wife, Stephanie. We have all lived active and fulfilled lives, including Krystie. We haven't let her illness dominate our lives including her own. We have always shown great versatility in our ability to minimise the effect of Krystie's illness.

The majority of our family's ability to handle this situation has been down to my mom who went head first into finding ways to slow Krystie's condition. I think that she achieved this successfully. She did this whilst continuing to maintain a high-pressure career, bringing up two young children, and also keeping a watchful eye over us older ones. My mother's commitment to all these things has meant that we have all been compelled to keep moving forward in our lives.

When Krystie's illness was confirmed, Nicholas and I were told that we were to be tested for the condition. It seemed that it was possible that either one of us could have it too, but that the symptoms just hadn't started to show yet.

Nicholas was keen to be tested. Personally I didn't want to know. I didn't want my future taken away from me and I didn't know how I would handle a positive result. I preferred to wait and see if the symptoms emerged. I couldn't see myself having the will to continue if I had been struck by Friedreich's Ataxia too. This makes me feel cowardly; having watched Krystie develop her life so bravely, achieving both personal and academic success.

Nicholas and I took the blood test. They both returned negative – we are only carriers just like our parents. The emotions of those results were mixed. I was happy to be negative, but then also saddened and disgusted by the situation for Krystie. When you feel such emotions you question the purpose of life. We should all be on this earth to live a rich and fulfilled life. We should all be handed the same platform! How could it be fair that Krystie had the disease, and I didn't? It wasn't, it simply wasn't!

In my opinion you cannot reason in your mind something like Krystie's illness. It is just down to the cruelty of life, a cruelty that shouldn't exist.

As Krystie's condition has degenerated we have adjusted to each and every circumstance. Nothing has proved to be overly difficult for us to handle. This was until her back operation. In spring 2004 we were told Krystie was to have surgery on her back at some point within the following year. The risks of this operation were huge. For the first time we saw Krystie's life in danger! I felt scared; I didn't want to lose her. There was a point early on where I thought that this was a possibility. All the early indications were poor and there didn't seem much to be positive about. I went on a trip that was already planned of self-exploration in the summer of 2004; travelling in Australia and South East Asia. I went with Krystie's pending operation fresh in my mind. I had a truly wonderful summer but the whole time was tinged with sadness. I was experiencing the most amazing times, being involved in some truly fantastic activities and I didn't think that Krystie would ever experience these things too.

As the operation drew closer the prognosis wasn't so grim and by the actual day of her operation I felt quite positive that she was going to be 'okay'. I just didn't have the feeling that it was all going to go wrong; it just wasn't that time.

Even so, sitting in the hospital waiting room as the clock was ticking, and the operation time became longer and longer, I became nervous that something had indeed gone wrong. Then the doctor appeared. . . . I was on my way to the toilet so met him in the doorway. From the moment I saw his face I knew she was fine. You could see he was a man who had done a good day's work. His eyes sparkled and he greeted me with a smile.

'Are you the family of Krystie Maddox-Lue,' he said.

'Yes,' I replied.

'She's doing fine, she's in recovery, it's gone well!'

Just like that, nearly eighteen months of worry were over!

Krystie's illness continues, and so does life. Nobody knows what's around the next turn. Krystie continues to live a happy and fulfilled life. I think she is sometimes frustrated by her situation, which is understandable, but she still does a fantastic job in staying positive. Watching her live her life so bravely means that you only have one choice and that is to enjoy yours.

The future 14

I was glad to see the back of 2005. If we can survive that year, I'm sure we can survive anything!

Our family has experienced many things in the last few years. We have lived through highs and lows. We have all learnt that no matter how hard things are, you can actually get through them. We don't take anything for granted. All of us appreciate the delicate balance of life. I think that on the whole, we take time for each other. We love to do things as a family. Even my strapping 'big lads' are pleased enough to join in the family events, and they both 'look out' for Krystie. The whole experience has definitely brought us closer together.

We have faced many challenges, and I know that we have many more to come. We are not alone; it's true to say that most people have their own story to tell. What never ceases to amaze me is the human capacity to cope and rise above adversity. And you know, I do believe that challenges make us the people we are; they give us the insight and empathy to help others.

Krystie is the one whose life continually changes, yet she refuses to give up. She has regained her zest for life, and doesn't seem to worry about anything. She is approaching her examinations with determination. She is writing her stories, and has started to paint again. She has taken up wheelchair basketball (after all)! I think that her head has finally caught up with her body; she isn't wasting time being depressed, she just wants to do as much as she can. She has attended an audition for a new BBC drama series, and is hoping that she will be successful. Because she is disabled she can learn to drive at the age of 16, which she will be in

March (2006) so we are busy trying to sort out her lessons, and then an adapted car. I can't imagine her behind the wheel of a car, but she can't wait!

Physically her body seems to have regained some of its strength and she is able to stand with support for around five minutes, which is great because she really needs to maintain the ability to transfer between her wheelchair and her bed, or the toilet or the sofa. That one act of being able to stand for just a few minutes means a lot to her. Yes, she is doing really well. She is still Miss Independence, and tells me that she is hoping to buy her own apartment and move out when she's about 19. She makes me smile with her optimism and exuberance. What a lesson to us all. I am sure that she will achieve whatever she wants to. I will always be there in the background for her. I know that we can expect more physical changes over the years, but I also know that we will manage. I am convinced that her own mental attitude will always pull her through. So it's best to leave the future in front, and concentrate on now. I think that you need to live each day, and close it with no regrets. I obviously do think about Krystie a lot. She is my first thought in the morning, and my last thought at night. I think about that 'perfect' little girl who was handed to me fifteen years ago, and now know that medically she wasn't. But as I watch her greet each day without complaint, and tackle her life with determination, I have to say that she is as perfect as any of us with all our human frailties. I'm proud to have her; she is perfect, perfectly flawed.

Krystie

My future's full of uncertainty. Sometimes I worry that because of my illness I won't be able to do much for myself later on in life; that all my days of fun have been and gone. But I realise that actually that isn't true. There's always another happy day just around the corner. Life is so full of uncertainty, for everyone. No one knows what's in store for them, but we can't just stand still and hope nothing bad comes our way. Life is for the living, and I blatantly refuse to sit back and allow everyone else to move on without me. My life is moving quickly. Even now, I find myself wondering where the time has gone. I want a husband and children and things to change; and at the same time I want everything to stay as it is. I think everyone feels like that at some point, don't ask me why, I have no idea. But I do know one thing. Whatever happens, I won't waste a second of my life, not ever!

Useful contacts

Ataxia UK – 0845 644 0606
www.ataxia.org.uk

Contact a Family – 0808 808 3556
www.cafamily.org.uk

Integrated medical centre – 020 7224 5111
www.integrated.med.co.uk

Childlife – 01252 628 072
www.childlife.org.uk

Krystie's blog
www.myspace.com/Krystie_123